TELEMEDICINE SERVICES

AN ARGUMENT FOR USE IN AFRICAN, HAITIAN, & U.S. VIRGIN ISLANDS HEALTHCARE SYSTEMS

DR. HUGUES FIDELE BATSIELILIT, PH.D
PUBLIC HEALTH SPECIALIST

Telemedicine Services: An Argument for use in African, Haitian, & U.S. Virgin Islands Healthcare Systems

All Rights Reserved

Copyright © 2021 by Hugues Batsielilit

No part of this book may be reproduced or transmitted, downloaded, distributed, reverse engineered, or stored in or introduced into any information storage and retrieval system, in any form or by any means, including photocopying and recording, whether electronic or mechanical, now known or hereinafter invented without permission in writing from the publisher.

The contents of this work, including but not limited to, the accuracy of events, people, and places depicted; opinions expressed; permission to use previously published materials included and any advice given, or actions advocated, are solely the responsibility of the author, who assumes all liability for said work and indemnifies the publisher against any claims stemming from the publication of the work.

Please send all correspondence to:
The International Consulting Aid Network (ICAN)
609 Gravlee Lane
Birmingham, Alabama, 35206

DEDICATION

I dedicate this book to the men and women of the healthcare industry who work diligently to make Telemedicine technology available to Africa and the Caribbean, specifically the U.S. Virgin Islands (USVI) and Haiti.

Dr. Hugues Fidele Batsielilit, Ph.D.

ACKNOWLEDGMENTS

Telemedicine Services: An Argument for Use in African, Haitian, and U.S.Virgin Islands Healthcare Systems is the shared achievement of countless specialists and partners from various countries, who worked with me toward a common idea that Telemedicine technology must be incorporated into the health systems of Africa, the USVI, and Haiti. Their dedication to gathering and sharing the information necessary to create this work, powered the conviction to push forward with what proved to be a challenging project.

My heartfelt acknowledgment extends to the Review Team which, under the chairwomanship of Karen Stafford, identified innovative approaches to assure the production of a reliable book within an environment hindered by limitations of two essential resources: time and money.

Special recognition to other professional colleagues who committed their time and suggestions to this publication including, my lovely daughter, Froy Moussavou Batsielilit.

AUTHOR

Dr. Hugues Fidele Batsielilit, Ph.D., is the President and CEO of the International Consulting Aid Network (ICAN). He currently works as an emergency management specialist focusing on health, public health issues, and post-disaster impacts (Federal Emergency Management Agency), served as an expert international consultant in public health surveillance, a communicable disease specialist (The Peace Corps, and ICAN), a healthcare administrator, and a community health coordinator for more than ten years.

Batsielilit received his Bachelor of Science degree from the National Institute of Executives, a Master of Sciences and a Ph.D. in public health and healthcare administration from the University of Phoenix in Arizona. Additionally, Dr. Batsielilit holds an associate degree in medical logistics from the Fort Lee Military Academy in Virginia. He served in the United States Army from 2008 to 2012, where he was assigned to the 82nd Airborne Medical Division as a medical logistics specialist.

Dr. Batsielilit is a member of several professional associations, including the Army Medical Veterans, the Peace Corps RPCV, the Nonprofit Association of Alabama, the Red Cross, the Birmingham Chamber of Commerce, the British Council, and the American College of Healthcare Executives.

TABLE OF CONTENTS

Telemedicine Services: An Argument for Use in African, Haitian, and U.S. Virgin Islands Healthcare Systems

Introduction xi

Chapter One... 1
    Part 1: State of Public Healthcare
    Services in African countries, the USVI, and Haiti.................. 3
    Part 2: Inefficiencies in the existing
    healthcare systems contributing to disparities 17
    Poor Governance... 21
    Inadequate and Inefficient Health Systems 23
    The Healthcare Financing Process............................... 27
    Counterfeit drugs in the healthcare systems 28
    Shaping the Future of Health in
    African Countries the USVI, and Haiti........................... 30

Chapter Two: Overview of Telemedicine 33
    Part 1: Definition of Telemedicine 35
    Five major benefits of telemedicine:............................. 36

Four main modalities used for Telemedicine. 37
Part 2: Origin and global history of telemedicine usage 39
Part 3: Components and systems needed to implement telemedicine . . .41
Part 4: Literature evaluation approach 43
Evaluation Benchmarks. 43
Part 5: Benefits of telemedicine to
improving access and healthcare quality 47
Telemedicine closes the gap in specialty referrals 52
Telemedicine aims to avoid unnecessary emergency room visits 52
Healthcare providers benefit from Telemedicine platforms 53
Remote and rural communities'
benefit from Telemedicine's accessibility 54
Part 6: The role of Telemedicine in improving
medical education or continuing education for providers. 57
Telemedicine Services in a Healthcare Context. 60

Chapter Three: Bringing Telemedicine to Africa, Haiti, and the USVI . . . 67
Part 1: Telemedicine pilot projects in Africa, Haiti, and the USVI. . . . 69
Part 2: Implementing Telemedicine
today in Africa, Haiti, and the USVI 75
External impediments to achieving improved health care systems. . . 79
Healthcare Provider Engagement 80
Health system challenges 85
Training 89
Ensuring sustainability 90
Reimbursement challenges
through public and private insurance entities. 91

Chapter Four: Additional Applications of Telemedicine 95

    Part 1: Healthcare provider shortage. 97

    Part 2: Health sub-specialties that
add value in healthcare provider shortage 101

Chapter Five: Telemedicine, Politics, and Regulations 131

Chapter Six: Looking Forward: Emerging Risks 135

    Part 1: Emerging technological risks. 137

    Part 2: Emerging technological risks: Avoiding Fraud Schemes 141

    Part 3: Emerging health risks: new infectious diseases
and how they may affect or lead to changes in telemedicine 147

Chapter Seven: Future of Telemedicine 151

Conclusion. 153

Recommendations 157

INTRODUCTION

The continual absence of reliable governance and the relentless curse of poverty keep African countries and Haiti from providing effective access to quality health services. More than most nations of the world, Haiti and many countries on the African continent continue to endure persistent resurgence of infectious diseases, rises in chronic illness burden, and other medical anomalies, which are principal threats to their people. [1,2,3] Added to the prevalence of disease is the difficulty in accessing quality care which has become a nationwide outcry as citizens contend with poor services in the public sector and unaffordable medical expenses from private facilities.

The current struggle is how to provide populations with quality, accessible healthcare, and achieve comprehensive coverage without incurring economic adversity. Much of the inadequacy of existing health systems is due in part to inefficiencies in staff retention and education, difficulties acquiring equipment, and problems with equipment maintenance and repair. Further, a critical shortage of healthcare providers, comingled with profound budgetary limitations which affects proper hospital facility governance, government ineptitude, corruption, misappropriation, and/or mishandling of funds and income inequities affect all aspects of health and health services.

Reinforcing these problems are government policies which foster corruption rather than integrity thereby, contributing to endemic health disparities despite increases in many of the governments' budgets. Together, these factors are a strident call for innovative approaches to improve current healthcare disruption.[4]

Research to find information about the state and quality of healthcare in the U.S. Virgin Islands was difficult as very little scholarly published work is available. The majority of the documents discussing health in the USVI tend to be national surveys such as the Behavioral Risk Factor Surveillance System (BRFSS). A singular study funded by a three-year grant to the National Institutes of Health National Center on Minority Health and Health Disparities (NIH/NCMHD) allowed the nursing program at the University of the Virgin Islands to set up a program focusing on health disparities and provide support to the University to investigate the issues. The program that was established by the grant was the Caribbean Exploratory Research Center (CERC).

The study found that, similar to African nations and Haiti, residents of the island feel that the quality of care is lacking, equipment is not properly maintained, and there are questions surrounding medical education, the qualifications of healthcare providers, and the protection of personal and health information. These factors are exacerbated by exorbitant costs, along with major gaps in accessibility to quality care between wealthier off-islanders (from the U.S. mainland) who have retired to the islands or spend winters there, and inhabitants whose families have resided there for generations. [5]

Telemedicine technology has enormous potential to minimize some of the challenges faced by these nations. The platform can overcome geographic boundaries and broaden access to health care services for rural and disadvantaged communities. In light of this potential, the book examines the benefits Telemedicine services can bring to health care and a populations' welfare.

Included in this work are suggested telemedicine solutions which can be implemented at the national, regional, and international levels. Additional discussions on how the technology can provide African countries, the USVI, and Haiti's healthcare providers and stakeholders with reliable information and management best practices, strategies, and standards in telemedicine implementation are also a part of this body of work.

The use of existing internet-based communications such as e-mail, medical web portals, and upgrading current top-speed capacity to conduct healthcare services and provide teleconsultations, are encouraging aspects upon which to move forward and begin telemedicine projects.

Many factors can affect telemedicine's adoption and practice; however, assessments revealed there is great acceptance of the value of this technology and a willingness to work to overcome difficulties that might be incurred in carrying out its implementation. Based on data from the Telemedicine field assessment and meetings, several thematic areas, as well as approaches that simplify the promotion and prompt improvement of telemedicine services, were evaluated and refined to form this book.

We cannot overestimate the seriousness of assessment within the field of telemedicine. The technology is in its infancy and while its potential is vast, evaluation can ensure maximization of benefits.

While African countries, the USVI, and Haiti may be more prone to view resource issues such as costs, weak infrastructure, and shortage of specialized expertise to be roadblocks to telemedicine implementation, our recommendations are further reasons to consider the benefits telemedicine technologies will grant to any existing healthcare operations experiencing the myriad of problems listed herein.

Telemedicine will not resolve all health system difficulties confronting these countries. The technology can however, help decrease, and in some cases ameliorate, exorbitant pricing of medical care services and other obstacles to accessibility and the actual delivery of quality care. The platform can also improve the clinical experience by allowing for more focused clinical interviewing, emergency evaluations, and other one-on-one medical services wherein conversations between the clinician and the patient or their family member(s) needs to take place. This technology will allow for the creation of healthcare services in country sides and/or rural areas where distance affects accessibility.

Therefore, African countries, the USVI, and Haiti's governments should take advantage of the capacity of telemedicine platforms by forming specialized agencies to harmonize telemedicine actions, assuring they comply with local, national, and international standards, are cost-effective, and are assessed and financed as part of overall coordinated healthcare service delivery.

Government representatives, healthcare providers, NGOs, and community representatives, to name just a few, should be reminded telemedicine technology brings medicine back into communities and individual homes. Therefore, they should see telemedicine as a competitive edge for healthcare providers and physician practices rather than as a competitor to existing services and platforms.

However, while the prospect of incorporating and implementing Telemedicine platforms within African countries, the USVI, and Haiti's healthcare systems is exciting and promising, it is also important to be mindful of the limitations of this book, the most significant of which was the struggle to get data sources of the best quality and accessible references.

In past decades, we have seen a slight improvement in healthcare data-collection processes in a few African countries; however, some data collected, especially those related to Telemedicine services in Haiti, were not precise or practical. To avoid bias in the data gathered, we have tried to provide the most references possible. A concession of this work is the data sources and references offered might not be current and may therefore, underline the need to improve data-gathering systems related to healthcare information for knowledgeable decision-making.

It is possible the countries of focus in this book may have incorporated and implemented some suggested Telemedicine platforms and taken effective measures targeting long-term sustainability for the well-being of their populations. However, of utmost importance is that governments continue prioritizing the incorporation of telemedicine services into existing health systems and promoting the collection and analysis of data that will allow accurate reporting on the services that have and will be disbursed and those in usage.

CHAPTER ONE

PART 1:
STATE OF PUBLIC HEALTHCARE SERVICES IN AFRICAN COUNTRIES, THE USVI, AND HAITI

The current public health systems are in a continuous crisis-state manifested in disrupted systems largely due to defeated and ineffective leadership and poor governance, which have resulted in systems and administrations wherein corruption usually rules. A demand for equitable access to quality health services has become a nation-wide outcry from the populations of these nations as they contend with poor services in the public sector and/or unaffordable medical expenses from private health facilities.

In African countries, the USVI, and Haiti, the highest disparities in healthcare delivery are in primary care and medical specialties, especially those whose focus is chronic illness. Most of the services provided in these two medical areas are generally offered through the public-health system (government), the rest by private health facilities (privately funded), including nonprofit organizations, and traditional healers. Primary care delivered in the public sector in some African countries is free and can be provided at no cost to specific populations in the USVI and Haiti. However, private, and nonprofit organizations often charge out-of-pocket fees.

Two types of facilities deliver public primary-care services in these countries: Hospitals and public or private health centers/clinics, with hospitals usually being the largest medical centers with the greatest varieties of clinical facilities for patient care, basic science, and translational research

Hospitals tend to have sufficient land space to house or the ability to fund the physical association of other medical establishments such as specialty institutions, medical schools, nursing, dentistry, public health, and pharmacy schools along with other health-related practices.[6] Public or private health centers, however, are community-based, patient-directed organizations that provide broad, primary health care services.[7] Health centers often integrate access to pharmacy, mental health, substance use disorder, and oral health services in localities where economic, geographic, or cultural barriers limit access to affordable health care services.[8] Such extensive health systems provide care to extremely vulnerable populations, especially those living in remote and rural areas. Despite the services provided by these health structures, primary care and access to quality care remains insufficient and challenging for most of the population.[9,10]

As of today, healthcare organizations in many African countries, the USVI, and Haiti are trailing other developing countries in health care improvements and outcomes and are thus undermining the well-being of their populations.[11] Another factor of significance is that the abyss between rich and poor is greater than ever, further exacerbating disparities in accessibility, affordability, and quality of care.

In many African countries, the prevailing state of healthcare structures is far from adequate and applicable health infrastructure is unusable and constrained because of countless individuals relying on it. Most public run healthcare structures in urban and rural areas are often clustered, lack vital drugs, incur persistent shortages of necessary medications, and tend to have suboptimal treatment and prescription use. Added to these issues is a lack of storage facilities for pharmaceutical products, unethical procurement processes, limited availability of beds, and often outdated technology and equipment. While this is the case for many metropolitan areas in African countries and Haiti, and some of the facilities in the USVI, according to annually published reviews conducted by global-growing.org and worldometers.info, 63 percent of the population, especially in Africa, live in rural areas without access to proper sanitation systems, hygiene, clean water, and basic healthcare services. A report conducted by the WHO added that in 2013, the African continent, especially sub-Saharan Africa, had a deficit of over 1.8 million healthcare providers and this was expected to increase to over 4.3 million by 2035. Just a few countries have emphasized the desire to build modern hospitals or reform existing ones to reduce the distance for access to quality healthcare services. The lack of funding resources reinforces the challenges associated with quality healthcare infrastructure continuing to undermine the delivery of care services offered by hospitals and health centers.

A report by the International Finance Corporation (IFC) (2007) comments that African countries command less than 1% of international health spending and have only 3 percent of the globe's health care workforce. Yet, Africa as a continent, accounts for "almost half" the deaths of children under age 5 globally, continues to have the world's highest maternal mortality rate, and has the greatest proportion of people living with HIV/AIDS and malaria. All these factors coalesce to help create an enormous financial loss in healthcare infrastructure and delivery.[12] Further, the African continent is shown to have an average physician density of 0.19 doctors per 1000 people which translates to barely one physician for every 5000 persons.[13] This critical shortage of healthcare providers undoubtedly causes harm with significant consequences to overall healthcare services, and also affects the enthusiasm of the few remaining healthcare providers to continue serving beyond the call of duty. The nonexistence of adequate healthcare structures and the shortage of certified, licensed professional healthcare providers, especially in inaccessible and remote areas, has resulted in populations seeking relief and treatment from traditional health workers and healers.

As of today, the steadfast motivation of healthcare providers is being outpaced by political priorities and insufficient financial allocations for healthcare systems. On the frontline of a population's survival, many physicians are overburdened, overstressed, and working without the assistance they need. Many are failing under the burden, and others are pursuing a better living and more rewarding work in developed countries. A newly published study financed by the Gates Foundation found that migration to developed countries is the number one cause of loss of healthcare specialists.[14] The shortage has further unforeseen impacts upon rural populations manifested in increased loss of critical primary and preventive care physicians which exacerbates disparities in access and quality of care for rural and non-rural areas.

Further, disease and mortality rates for infants, children, and expectant mothers are increasing as urban and rural areas experience decreasing numbers of less than one doctor per thousand persons according to a 2004 Rockefeller Foundation report.[15] Much of this is a direct repercussion of governments' incapacity to re-energize the healthcare structures, especially in inaccessible localities, resulting in high child and maternal mortality rates, low newborn birth weights, poor sanitation, and overall excessively inadequate healthcare access.[16] As of today, constructive approaches to remedy the health workforce shortage in African countries remains limited.

More telling than statistics on the numbers of physicians and healthcare specialists Africa lacks is the fact that according to the United Nations World Mortality Report, the African continent has the highest mortality rates, and it is the only continent where deaths from infectious diseases still outnumber deaths from chronic illnesses.[17-19] Coupled with this troubling fact it is also reported that half of the 10 million children who die worldwide below the age of five are in Africa and they die from lack of access to healthcare services, high levels of poverty, malaria, and malnutrition.[20] The reports further claim that undeveloped infrastructure and poor conditions in health facilities contribute to deaths of children when born or those in need of medical help.[21]

In addition to insufficient funding, the healthcare systems are affected by persistent corruption in the public healthcare sector. Despite minor improvements in campaigns to alter or even stop this nefarious activity, the incidence remains high in the majority of African nations. Ongoing corruption deflects considerable-needed resources away from health care delivery and limits access to quality care services for those entire populations, especially those residing in rural and remote areas.

In its yearly Global Corruption report, Transparency International identified the African health sector as corruption-prone with proof of inducement across the entire scope of health services. The report further asserts that corruption is persistent throughout the public healthcare sector.[22-25]

Corruption among actual healthcare providers – physicians, nurses, medical technicians, etc. is systemic and can mean the difference between life and death for those needing medical care. In its Periodical Corruption report, Stanford Business Education contends that healthcare providers within African public health care facilities have been selling medications that should be free of charge and are diverting other medicines and supplies for private sector resale.[26, 27]

Along with these issues, the area having the most significant consequences is that of inadequate healthcare funding. This singular factor has widespread, overarching impact affecting education of healthcare providers, maintenance of existing healthcare systems and physical structures, creation of needed healthcare infrastructure, incorporation of new technologies such as telemedicine, maintenance, repair, and purchase of necessary equipment, and many other components that make up all that is vital to healthcare delivery. Added to the shortcomings of the aforementioned challenges and problems, is that resistance to prioritize and therefore fund healthcare and healthcare systems so they are viable and sustainable, creates an undue economic burden across weak and poor-income groups. Effective investments in public health continue to be reduced and/or redirected to other non-pressing matters. Added to all of this is the fact that health facilities lack proper data collection procedures, which makes monitoring, evaluation, implementation and tracking of quality control performance measures challenging and difficult to improve.

Changes to this entire system can be achieved in several ways:

- Increased and equitable pay for all healthcare workers would provide incentives for them to remain in the field.
- Structured and monitored oversight of healthcare worker and physician certifications,
- Monitored oversight of pharmaceuticals and pharmacy staff
- The establishment of medication protocols for distribution, handling, and storage
- Government budgets that include targeted increased spending initiatives on healthcare coupled with accountability measures for oversight of allocation and distribution of funds.

Changes such as these would result in significant, visible, and tangible changes and improvement throughout the healthcare systems of Haiti, the USVI, and even Africa.

For Haiti and African nations another factor that would benefit health care services would be if government administrations would establish a fully regulated, true insurance system that is affordable and provides incentives for users to practice preventive health and to maintain health through exercise, medication information, and health and nutrition education programs. Disenfranchised and rural, as well as impoverished and underpaid urban populations, would benefit from these improvements if mandated and actually implemented. All the aforementioned have the propensity, when performed and implemented with careful oversight, to result in improved systems of health care and an improved health outcomes.

The Caribbean region, including the USVI and Haiti, have similar public health concerns and contend with some of the same major threats of infectious diseases every year as effective public health surveillance programs are not implemented.

❖ Regarding Haiti, however, it is not an overstatement to say that the 2010 earthquake that all but demolished the small nation, set its healthcare facilities (hospitals, clinics, and health centers) on a course back to a medically primitive era.

The earthquake caused damage to health care structures and cut off or caused the shut-down of essential critical services for the delivery of health care including the electrical grid, transportation, water, and sanitation systems.[28] The nation's leading teaching hospital, clinical and trauma referral center, L'Hôpital Université d'Etat d'Haïti (Haitian State University Hospital or HUEH), was damaged and lost two-thirds of its structures in the 2010 earthquake, and is yet in a disastrous condition.[29]

As of today, the Haitian government has organized the health care delivery system into three levels: primary care provided at some health centers and community hospitals; departmental hospitals which offer secondary care; and university hospitals and specialized centers which deliver tertiary care. Of more than 900 health establishments, 38% are public, 42% are private, and

20% are integrated. [30-31] Granted, Haiti's health sectors have had encouraging improvements in some fields, however, significant stagnation in separate sectors remains to be resolved. These diverse issues reveal a health sector that repeatedly faces significant challenges.[32]

One medical improvement accredited to the focus on rebuilding the HUEH is the Tuberculosis clinic which operated under tents after the earthquake, is now housed in a building. The TB treatment center was established in 2010 by US volunteer, Dr. Coffee, and a group of Haitian nurses. More than 1,000 TB patients have received treatment at the center since its inception.[33]

Monetary and geographical factors are other important challenges to accessing quality healthcare services in Haiti. Today, public and private healthcare facilities (93 percent) impose consultation fees. Although health services are, on most occasions, supported by the government, individuals are still obliged to pay fees for the services and supplies including gloves, syringes, and drugs. Public transportation is severely limited and impedes the ability of people to access health services, especially women ages 15–49 who travel for obstetric, gynecological, pediatric exams for their children. These factors further handicap the poorest populations in their efforts to receive effective health services.[34, 35]

In terms of infrastructure and its impact, work, living conditions, and in-patient accommodations for health providers and patients at public and private healthcare facilities have seen continual deterioration over several consecutive decades. Operationally, most medical equipment is not properly maintained and serviced, causing providers to work with machines that are damaged and/or in need of repair; emergency and operating rooms are not clean, and electrical failure is an ordinary occurrence even during surgical procedures.

Dispensaries, the foremost provider of outpatient healthcare services, are also among the most ineffective category of health facilities in Haiti compared with developing countries, according to the World Bank organization. Some dispensaries are street-side purveyors of expired and illicit medications purchased by people residing in overcrowded city slums, refugee camps, and rural areas. These are not regulated or monitored by any health or government authorities. There are some exceptions wherein private non-profits have established dispensaries that are manned by trained health workers and a physician is available for consultation; however, these are few and far between.[36]

It has been shown that public and private healthcare facilities (hospitals and dispensaries) lack effective internal management and accountability procedures. The domino effect of this is that healthcare providers have an unwillingness to apply effective clinical practice guidelines for quality primary and palliative care delivery.

Presently, Haiti lacks sufficient numbers of hospitals. This is a direct result of the significant shortfall in public expenditures upon the healthcare system. The Haitian government spends most health funds on curative, rather than preventive care. This spending formula results in excessive cost to patients, the nation, and increases demand on the system.[37,38]

Further, a sizeable amount of the funds spent on Haiti's public health facilities does not translate into substantial increased or improved capacity of service delivery. Even though expenses appear to be significant in unequivocal terms, the funds available for hospitals are insufficient compared to countries such as the Dominican Republic and Cuba which allocate a substantial amount on public health.[39, 40]

According to "Better Spending, Better Care: A Look at Haiti's Health Financing", a report from the World Bank (2017), "the annual per capita public health spending in Haiti is $13, compared with $781 in nearby Cuba and $180 in the Dominican Republic, Haiti's neighbor on the island of Hispaniola.

Public investment in health care has plummeted from 16.6 percent of the total Haitian government budget in 2004."[41]

The Haitian government funds a fraction of overall health disbursement, non-budgetary, and directs it through many facilitators. Further, significant lack of proven standardized procedures for technical and financial donations has been undermining public health delivery effectiveness.[42] In February 2014, to restructure its finances, Haitian President, Michel Martelly, asked that the United States change the way it sent aid money to Haiti, calling for it to funnel more through the government rather than non-governmental organizations (NGOs). Martelly acknowledged that the reason for distributing money through NGOs had been 'corruption' in Haiti and 'lack of confidence in the Haitian system'.[43]

Targeted allocations for health systems and programs assure sustainability, affordability, and social protection by providing for the health of the nation's populous. However, the continuous decrease of fiscal resources to the health sector adds more burden to the prevalent health care systems.

With a contingent of 3.5 health professionals per 10,000 residents, the doctor to patient ratio in Haiti is 4 times below the smallest standard set forth by the World Health Organization (WHO) of 25 doctors per 10,000 population. [44-46] Due to reduced funding sources at the national level, public healthcare facilities are experiencing an unprecedented shortage of doctors. Approximately 40% of healthcare providers, educated in Haiti, either left the field of medicine or are emigrating abroad to countries such as the US, Canada, and South America for better opportunities.[47]

Corruption is another variable affecting Haiti's healthcare system. It creates and contributes to financial drain and negative health service results. Transparency International's Corruption Perception Index for 2008 ranked Haiti as the fourth most corrupt country in the world.

Health corruption in the public and private healthcare systems has been severe for years and is an unprecedented impediment to the country's health efforts in resource-poor settings, and drains resources from the already delicate health systems, limiting access to quality health service for the most defenseless and needy people.[48, 49]

Haiti's public health systems are believed to be lacking in clarity, monitoring control, and the implementation and enforcement of effective mandated regulatory policies which creates an environment ripe for and with extortion and bribes, and the sale of fake and expired medicines. Present corruption risks in the healthcare systems also include the diversion of funding resources resulting in fraud, theft, and the misallocation of budgets. [50-51]

While the United States Virgin Islands are far away from Haiti, the two share similar aspects related to the impacts and aftereffects of disaster and the slow progress of recovery processes. The USVI covers 346 square miles, with a population projection of more than 104,456 people according to several published reports including the 2010 U.S. Census, living mainly on three islands: St. Croix, St. Thomas, and St. John.[52,53] More than two years after two major hurricanes (Irma and Maria) struck the U.S. Virgin Islands, the effects of the storms on the healthcare systems are still noticeable. Although portions of the health care systems have resumed activities, gaps, and inequitable services remain significant. The territory's hospitals on St. Croix, St. John, and St. Thomas continue to cope with substantial infrastructure damage and reductions in serviceability.[54] Both the primary hospitals, Schneider Regional Medical Center on St. Thomas and Governor Juan F. Luis Hospital on St. Croix, some urgent care centers, clinics, and health department facilities experienced damages that limit their ability to provide full services.[55,56] Government leaders have determined it could take up to twenty-four months to either improve or replace the Schneider Regional Medical Center facility.

According to several published sources, the USVI governor's office has indicated the desire that both hospitals be destroyed and reconstructed.[57]

In the absence of healthcare facilities, an additional major challenge is the shortage of healthcare providers, many of whom left the islands after the storms, emigrating mainly to the United States because of damages to their own homes and for better opportunities.

Adding to the hardships, is the financial crisis healthcare facilities are confronting as they struggle under the budgetary burden of uncompensated care, decreased, or eliminated profit opportunities, and limited Government assistance, all of which cause further decreases in the delivery and effectiveness of health services and patient flow. As a result of all these inadequacies and deficiencies, people with health insurance have been forced to pursue substitute health services stateside or in nearby Puerto Rico. In addition, insurance premiums and deductibles have increased while providing limited coverage, resulting in further pushing the outward migration in search of adequate healthcare.

Although the health care systems in the United States Virgin Islands appear not to be in as dire straits as those in Haiti, there are many parallels between the health conditions of the populations sharing similar living situations.[58]

Aside from dissimilarities in size and population combined with geographic and practical remoteness, the unembellished economic limitations, scarcity of medical equipment and vital medicines, including diminishing physical amenities, and inefficiencies in improvement and abilities, communication structures, and technical and organizational infrastructure, the USVI presents the same deficits and problems.

As of today, infectious diseases (whether new, persistent, or recurring) are a substantial problem and remain a considerable peril to African nations and Haiti. As part of the Sustainable Development Goals, the World Health

Organization countries agreed to achieve free universal health coverage (UHC) by 2030. As of January 2019, all the United Nations (UN) member-states, which includes thirty-five African nations, Haiti, and the USVI (as a non-self-governing territory) agreed to implement UHC by the WHO deadline. However, according to WHO findings during COVID-19, member-state nations have failed, and are failing in meeting the sustainable goals to which they agreed. [50]

Universal health care is a critical component of accessible healthcare. The lack of UHC causes access to equitable and good healthcare services to remain an ever- present social, economic, and political issue, is a major deterrent to people – especially the poor – seeking needed care.

Overall, however, governments and healthcare policymakers of these countries have assumed little responsibility for assuring equitable access to quality health services for their entire populations. Sadly, this posture of failure speaks to the unwillingness of these governments to enact legislation and policies, to take necessary steps to bring about improvements in existing healthcare infrastructure and systems, and to build new ones that are more efficient and effective for the delivery of better health outcomes.[60] A direct result of this inaction and prevailing ineptitude is that millions of poor people are forced into life-threatening hardship incurring exorbitant out-of-pocket healthcare expenditures. Joint news released by the WHO and the World Bank emphasizes that the poor generally devote over 10% per year of their family resources on "out-of-pocket" healthcare expenses.[61, 62] Therefore, ensuring a fair approach to both insurance and healthcare services calls for a transformation in how health benefits are subsidized, maintained, and allocated so that services are centered on the needs of people and communities that cannot afford basic and expensive care.

PART 2:
INEFFICIENCIES IN THE EXISTING HEALTHCARE SYSTEMS CONTRIBUTING TO DISPARITIES

It is important to note that many of the challenges faced by the healthcare systems of the nations focused upon in this book are long-standing and have heightened over the last 30 years. The conditions have always been acknowledged as deteriorating, fragile, and not operational, despite continual economic development. The provisional delivery healthcare in place remains basic, inefficient, and inappropriate.

Despite strong overall increases in budgets and monetary additions from national resources and international funding, the vast majority of the populations remain extremely impoverished, with substantial health disparities between rich and poor.[63, 64] Several published reports disclose that poverty and inequality between rich and poor persist causing an enduring, relentless social undertone.[65-67]

Per the World Health Organization's annual report, health disparities are mushrooming in many countries, contributing to the broadening social gap between the rich and the poor.[68]

The poor sometimes receive health services in abandoned and failing clinics and hospitals, while the richest, including heads of state, seek better medical services at top hospitals in foreign countries. It is further reported that many of the poor die because of ineffective health services and a shortage of qualified healthcare practitioners.[69, 70]

The reality, however, is that healthcare systems in these nations are not constructed with the wealthy in mind as few of them avail themselves of these often antiquated and inefficient systems. This fact emphasizes the significant gap between rich and poor: the impoverished are consigned to suffer in precarious and crippled hospitals which are yet striving to offer essential care services.

Poverty in Africa, and Haiti therefore, "has developed into a legitimized social condition that is illustrated by the absence of resources needed for basic existence".

The aforementioned statement is made in light of evidence which thoroughly substantiates and demonstrates that a vast majority of the populations of Africa and the nations of USVI and Haiti continue to live in a state of perpetual poverty further worsened by governments that ignore them except as they prove of political and financial benefit. They are disparaged and exist as underclass citizens. A glance at history reveals that people have only very infrequently contested inequality because they were led to believe that their inferior status in terms of income, wealth, and privilege was just, that it was not so bad, or that it was necessary for their future wellbeing. Ideological systems legitimized a status quo of inequality, and in more modern times, increasing inequity.[71, 72] Impediments to financial prosperity for the impoverished majority and degradation in their work conditions along with limitations of public health services allows these inequities to be perpetuated, leading to ever widening gaps.

The World Bank Organization, in its annual report, Accelerating Poverty

Reduction, explains how most countries with substantial poverty rates do not spend adequate financial resources on programs to decrease poverty, nor do they allocate funding resources in areas essential to the well-being of vulnerable populations.[73] Decreasing poverty-related to the financial and economic gap could be accomplished by devoting more targeted funding to the needs of poor communities.[74] Until then, endless discrepancies and disparities will continue to impact the concept of healthcare being delivered from a caring, social purpose perspective, provided through universal access as a social duty, to that of a profit-driven personal enterprise operated by immoral healthcare providers and corrupt authorities responsible for governance and accountability. These "immoral behaviors" lead to a population that is and has been unenthusiastic about seeking medical service, knowing they cannot receive the healthcare they deserve because of the presence of corruption in the healthcare systems.[75]

As of today, populations in these areas have become mindful that as soon as they reach a healthcare facility, they will have to pay expensive out-of-pocket expenses for services, even though funding is allocated for this purpose. [76] The World Health Organization periodic report claims that "out-of-pocket payments for health can cause households to incur catastrophic expenditures, which can push them into poverty. Key to protecting people is to ensure prepayment and pooling of resources for health, rather than relying on people paying for health services out-of-pocket at the time of use."[77]

It must be mentioned again that one of the most significant contributing factors to the problems and issues so far mentioned, is corruption in funding distribution and oversight of the healthcare systems. While expenditures amount to several billion US dollars, blatant corruption hinders that money from being useful and attainable across all facets of health care services sectors.[78]

Corruption, as defined by Transparency International and the World Bank, is: "the abuse of entrusted power or public office for private gain."[79] It is no mystery that the use of power and influence by health providers, representatives, and corporations for self-enrichment conflicts with their public responsibilities.

It is unfortunate that in many African nations, the USVI, and Haiti, health providers, representatives, and corporations have been exploiting current loopholes related to weak policies, absence of accountability, information disparities between healthcare providers, patients and suppliers, and public representatives for private gain. [80-82]

Embezzlement and resale of medicines are additional acts of corruption occurring at hospital delivery centers or government pharmaceutical resource centers.[83] In this context, universal access to primary health services is eroded with no signs of governments striving to correct the issues that further affect recovery and improvement. Although some degree of corruption can be found in all countries, its constant practice has been particularly devastating, especially for rural and remote locations in these places.

Health care professionals are entitled to fair wages for their labor, knowledge, skills, and the legitimate practice of medicine. The challenge remains to decrease pay inequity and gender discrimination along with bringing more prospects for underprivileged persons to have better lives. Overcoming these challenges, however, will necessitate all governments making concerted efforts to strive for improved community infrastructure, stable healthcare organizations, and the enactment and enforcement of funding and spending accountability measures.

Corruption and bribery are not the only determinants contributing to health inequities in the public health industry; additional significant factors have also been recognized to undermine the delivery of needed health services, particularly in remote and rural areas. Some of these are:

POOR GOVERNANCE

Governance plays a key role in the operation and performance of health systems. It can decrease disparities in health service quality if designed and implemented correctly. To define "governance," we rely on the definition from Kaufmann, Kraay, and Mastruzzi (2004, 2007): "the traditions and institutions by which authority in a country is exercised for the common good, which includes selecting those in authority, the capacity of the government to manage, and respect for the state."[84, 85] The World Health Organization expands this definition to include healthcare: "Governance in the health sector refers to a wide range of steering and rule-making related functions carried out by governments/decision-makers as they seek to achieve national health policy objectives conducive to universal health coverage."[86] Therefore, by definition, good governance in the healthcare industry is essential to increasing and improving performance in health care delivery.

Under tenets of good governance, the creation and enforcement of standards, the collection of information on performance, the leveraging of incentives for outstanding performance, quality, and accountability are required. Good governance can deter corruption, a significant consequence of poor governance that affects performance of the health sector and contributes to increased healthcare disparities. [87]

While the leadership of some developed countries use good governance as a strategy to build mechanisms that measure and support positive accomplishments to improve the wellbeing of the healthcare systems and the population, this is not the case in many African countries and Haiti. Oftentimes, countries lacking equitable and accessible quality health services have not made great improvements or investments in sustaining existing health systems and have not focused on planning good governance which could empower the population in their quest to gain access to basic healthcare services.[88, 89] The wellbeing of these countries depends, primarily, on the style of governance by which they implement decisions and strategize priority options to manage healthcare services. Governance comprises the use of political, economic, and administrative power to conduct public affairs and manage national resources.

Good governance has been demonstrated to result in positive social and economic outcomes. It inspires more strategic and targeted efforts toward achieving decided upon goals that will lead to desired improvements [90, 91] By comparison, the misuse of power, corruption, nepotism, and waste of limited public resources reduces a government's ability to offer good quality services to their population. As of today, poor governance accounts for much of the inefficiency in healthcare service delivery, and in certain situations results in no service at all. In such cases, governance is replaced by arbitrary policymaking, unaccountable bureaucracies, unenforced or unjust legal systems, and has led to economic disaster, corruption, political ambiguity, and unproductive regulatory laws and policies.

These issues contribute to health disparities and broaden the income gap. To reverse this trend, African nations, the USVI, and Haiti's governments need not only to eradicate the continued mishandling of public health resources, ensure quality service delivery and effective bureaucracy, and strengthen existing healthcare legislation, they must also strengthen accountability and transparency in the healthcare delivery systems.

INADEQUATE AND INEFFICIENT HEALTH SYSTEMS

As of today, health systems in many African countries, the USVI, and Haiti are not meeting the expectations related to delivery and access to quality care needed by their underprivileged populations. These healthcare systems have, over the past years, deteriorated from man-made or natural disasters, issues that cut across institutional, human resources, financial, technical, and political developments.

Evidence has shown that weak governance, human resource challenges, and financial impediments to healthcare services with high rates of out-of-pocket expenditures are connected to the ineffective integration of services in resource-limited nations.[92,93] Evidence also shows healthcare systems incapable of providing services in response to public health emergencies, such as an outbreak of infectious disease, leads to a rise in mortality and morbidity.

Despite increases in health budget expenditures, these countries have yet to achieve significant improvement in ensuring fairness in delivery. Expectations regarding healthcare services refers to the prospect or the certainty about what is being provided through the healthcare system. It is the subjective picture that the underprivileged population has of the process of communication with said systems.

Evidence of systemic healthcare inefficiencies is demonstrated in the health outcomes, mortality, and morbidity of the populations of these nations despite increases in health budget expenses. Mortality rates, which stand higher by international norms, have slightly decreased since 1990, but most of the improvement has happened among infants and the elderly.[94, 95] Although these countries' populations are living a little longer, the quality of life has not improved for people of working age, as self-reported health status continues to decrease among each age group.

One of the reasons inadequacy in healthcare system and healthcare access persist is because in many poorer nations governments manage public expectation downward. By consistently putting forth the message that there is a lack of adequate funds to improve services, and the insufficient numbers of qualified physicians is due to continual brain drain, the uneducated and poor, even when they do not believe their governments, cease to expect any changes in care and access and consistently accept terms and conditions that are unfavorable. Effects of unmet expectations can fluctuate from frustration to indignation, thereby further negatively affecting health.

Conversely, if governments accept, understand, and positively act on the expectations of the underprivileged, any recognition of those expectations or demonstration of affirmative change can result in improved health and psychological well-being, can reduce stress and its impacts on health.

In their current states, the health systems of these areas are trying to organize themselves around what patients need and focus on providing access to quality service to most of the population. Yet, they still are not accomplishing enough to lessen the burdening impact of illness on people's lives. Recurrent reductions in financial resources for healthcare continue to damage and aggravate the remaining fragile healthcare infrastructure, which makes services unavailable, inaccessible, high-priced, and uncontrolled. Medical providers in remote and rural locations often incur significant delays in receipt of clinical information, which further impedes the ability to deliver efficient and effective quality service.[96-100]

Currently, there has been limited emphasis on coordinating and improving investment in health infrastructure across these countries. As a result, these nations have a variety of types, quality, and functionality of infrastructure, making the assurance of delivering health service effectiveness and fairness challenging. Infrastructure, which includes the physical buildings, equipment, transport, and Information Communication Technology (ICT) requirements, necessitates coordinated strategy, maintenance, and continued upkeep and renovation.

The deteriorating condition of public health infrastructure and lack of motivation from authorities, are causes for concern to health workers in these countries. In certain locales, healthcare providers in public facilities (hospitals and clinics) have expressed disquiet over the poor conditions of the infrastructure, which they say has not been renovated or improved for the past decade, and many areas are overgrown by weeds.

Much of the infrastructure, besides deterioration, lacks essential equipment such as X-ray machines, chemistry machines or hematology analyzers, personal protective equipment (PPE), and COVID-19 training for healthcare providers.

Another factor affecting access to facilities is the lack of reliable transportation - whether public or private. The demand for proper transportation becomes greater when these resources are not accessible to the population. Ample evidence has established that transportation systems are a fundamental social element of health in rural and remote localities. Its accessibility allows vulnerable citizens the opportunity to access better health facilities and provide for additional care needs, purchase medications and nutritious food. Transportation systems herein are defined as any vehicle, activity, or other conveyance that carries people and goods from one place to another.

Major types of transportation include buses, trains, trucks, cars, airplanes, and other forms of motorized vehicles, such as boats and motorcycles, as well as non-motorized bicycles, and even pedestrian traffic.

Both public and private authorities manage transportation that may need preserving and modernizing of infrastructure to ensure fully operational and reliable systems. Evidence demonstrates that most of these countries' populations, especially those living in remote areas, do not access medical care due to transportation challenges. These barriers result in missed or delayed appointments and increased health expenses, which damages overall health.

Therefore, assuring access to essential health care services for vulnerable populations must include strategies and methods to ensure remediating inequities in service delivery, access, and quality are a priority. This assurance should be solidified by the existence and ready availability of adequate infrastructure and physical structures which includes trained staff, supplies, and equipment, and public infrastructure designed to sustain reliable transportation .

Governments and medical care organizations must engage vulnerable populations, establishing effective and trust-based relationships with them. Such engagement will form the backbone of interactions wherein people are active and informed participants in their healthcare and well-being. These collaborative efforts can lead to improved health outcomes and enable better and more rapid identification of problems and issues within the health system. However, enhancing access and value of care for vulnerable populations must also include improving current approaches to the use of scarce resources, and improving current communication and transportation systems and thereby accessibility especially for those living in rural and remote localities.

While these tasks may appear challenging, sufficient evidence and studies abound from which governments and health organizations may draw inspiration, ideas, and upon which feasible pragmatic solutions may be crafted. Specifically, there are viable examples of governments and health system leaders in developed countries shifting resources into areas outside critical sectors in order to satisfy the needs of their population, thereby improving health and health outcomes without increasing overall costs of services.

Overall, decreasing inequality and inefficiency in health systems in many African countries, the USVI, and Haiti will depend upon both enhancing approaches by which services are established and provided, and the creation of initiatives focusing on population health.

Simply put, inequality and inefficiency gaps cannot be decreased or closed without acting on the delivery of health care services and improving population health through public health efforts.

THE HEALTHCARE FINANCING PROCESS

Most African countries, the USVI, and Haiti still face a grim health scenario, particularly for those residing in distant localities. While some countries have seen limited progress in health improvements while chronic illnesses and infectious diseases remain high, and the health of the underprivileged continues to vacillate because of endless crises in the health financing process.

Healthcare financing systems are severely constricted by resource shortages and dependence on financial assistance from bilateral and multilateral contributors. This strategy leads to increased challenges in the provision of quality healthcare and contributes to high out-of-pocket expenditures for poor people.

According to the 2006 World Bank World Development Indicators Review, more than 50% of the populations of these countries lack access to improved healthcare infrastructure because of resource scarcity coupled with the high cost of health service.[101] Although the governments have pledged to allocate more money to healthcare, these promises remains unfulfilled.

To ease significant issues and impediments to quality healthcare, these governments need to support their healthcare industry improvement programs by funding them via mineral resources, taxes, and specific allocations based upon definitive population demographics and need. However, in environments wherein corruption is prolific, self-supported funding will be of little help if mismanagement of funds, insufficient allocations and distributions, and lack of accountability of how both government and the healthcare systems spend monies remain unresolved issues. In short, the development of standardized and strictly managed mechanisms for the oversight and equitable distribution of funds for health care are imperative if the health systems are to attain a level of adequacy that substantially meets the health needs of all populations of the nations addressed in this book.

COUNTERFEIT DRUGS IN THE HEALTHCARE SYSTEMS

Although, counterfeit drugs are not an unknown phenomenon in African countries, the USVI, and Haiti, their presence on the black market may have caused significant deaths among the population. As of today, the quantity of counterfeit drugs entering these countries is increasing and causing serious problems, especially for the underprivileged and those living in remote and rural areas as this may sometimes be their only recourse to access necessary medications.[102]

Throughout the world hundreds of thousands of counterfeit drugs slated to be destroyed or incinerated are instead, shipped to underdeveloped countries and distributed to black-markets. The supply and demand of black markets continues in the face of regulations and policies against such practices without regard for the health and safety of those forced to procure from such markets.

While it is impossible to quantify the real number and impact of these immense trafficking enterprises, the consequences to the public health industry and population continue to be destructive.

According to a World Health Organization (WHO) report, 1 in 10 drugs being prescribed or sold in these countries is deficient or counterfeit, and are causing the deaths of many people, primarily children.[103] It is asserted that the African continent alone claims more than 30% of counterfeit drugs in black market distribution.[104, 105] The continued distribution and sale of counterfeit medications and the public's painful familiarization with their ineffectiveness and death, has led to a broad mistrust of the public healthcare industry, including healthcare providers, the pharmaceutical industry, wholesalers, distributors, retailers, and government drug regulatory laws. A major consequence of the lack of trust is that those needing medications either do not purchase them when prescribed, or due to unaffordability, continue to patronize the black markets risking the onset of new illness, continued sickness, or death.

To better eradicate or decrease the supply and delivery of illicit drugs, targeted, and determined policies and enforcement from governments must be coordinated with all parties and implemented with consequences defined and carried out by the justice departments and law enforcement of these countries without leniency for the perpetrators. Another measure to contain and/or eradicate black market medication enterprises would be to establish and strengthen current collaboration with developed countries, private health, and community-based organizations to strategize actions that will ensure protection of the supply and distribution of medications.

Sharing data, information, establishing the identity of people involved in the trafficking, confiscating illicit drugs, medications, and medical supplies, incarcerating perpetrators, immediately destroying products, and enforcing punitive financial measures should be the highest priorities for all governments. Laws and regulations governing the sale and distribution of counterfeit and illicit pharmaceuticals should be made public along with guidance for how the public may report such crimes and knowledge of criminals without fear of retribution. A campaign of this type would have far-reaching impact if pharmaceutical establishments, healthcare providers, druggists, and the population at large are all informed and involved.

SHAPING THE FUTURE OF HEALTH

Holistic approaches to the healthcare systems of these nations is paramount not only for the remediation of the systems for the benefit of their people, but also for the treatment and eradication of persistent, resurgent infectious diseases and viruses because developing nations bear the brunt of the international health burden.[106-108] Less than 50% of the populations of these nations, especially those residing in rural and remote areas, have access to adequate, quality healthcare.[109, 110]

As mentioned in chapter one, the implementation of universal healthcare (UHC) would be one means of achieving more equitable and accessible healthcare. This would benefit both public and private sector healthcare systems.[111, 112] The inception of UHC is presently most promising in USVI and other Caribbean nations as those governments since 2018, have formed committees to collaborate on how to coordinate and then roll out UHC.[113]

In addition to UHC, the use of telemedicine technologies will further increase accessibility and equity: where UHC will help create a more expansive financial base wherein even the poorest will have more affordable access, telemedicine can open healthcare to the most rural populations via its broadband and internet-based platforms.[114, 115] Telemedicine technologies provide a significant alternative to traditional healthcare systems and are changing the way they deliver health services to poorer populations in rural and remote localities.

Telemedicine platforms give healthcare providers the ability to share through video conference and secure E-mails, patient records and data to help achieve better diagnostic results. Incorporating telemedicine technology within the health services setting has also been proven to support the cost-effectiveness of care delivery and extend the reach of services to remote locations. There is, however, little literature that speaks to the effectiveness of Telemedicine platforms and any improvement upon the quality of life and efficiency of health care services in African countries, and Haiti. In the USVI some health systems have initiated telemedicine services since the hurricanes (Irma and Maria) of 2018, and efforts are underway to expand services throughout the islands of the USVI.[116-118]

It is to the benefit of these countries, regardless of the absence of supporting data, to seize upon the power of Telemedicine, not only to bridge the rift in healthcare discrimination, but to also improve access to medical services. Though Telemedicine technology in these nations is still in the embryonic phase, incorporating and implementing the technology is viewed as a cost-effective approach to complement the current disrupted healthcare systems.

CHAPTER TWO:
OVERVIEW OF TELEMEDICINE

PART 1:
DEFINITION OF TELEMEDICINE

Telemedicine services are defined by the World Health Organization (2010), as *"The delivery of healthcare services, where distance is a critical factor, by all healthcare professionals using information and communication technologies for the exchange of valid information for the diagnosis, treatment, and prevention of disease and injuries, research and evaluation, and for the continuing education of healthcare providers, all in the interests of advancing the health of individuals and their communities."* [119]

While telemedicine technologies are applied to distant clinical applications through the use of communications infrastructure to deliver clinical services without in-person interaction, telehealth refers to a broad range of technologies and services such as providing medical education and training, managerial conferences, clinical services, surveillance, and health promotion.[120]

Both are significant, key components for creating and maintaining an effective effort to offer access to care and improve the effectiveness of healthcare delivery systems for most of the population, especially those living in rural and remote areas. However, for this book, telemedicine and telehealth will be used interchangeably.

FIVE MAJOR BENEFITS OF TELEMEDICINE:

1. Telemedicine technology can be used in far-flung areas and provided to masses of people.

2. It facilitates decision making allowing patient and physician to view and speak with one another and allows the physician to conduct assessments and diagnosis and to prescribe additional treatment regimens or medications.

3. It overcomes geographical boundaries, connecting individuals living in distant physical areas: communication can be achieved via wireless, internet, and other non-land bound technologies.

4. It uses many types of information and communication technologies thereby expanding methods of interaction and accessibility: Live video conferencing, mobile health apps, "store and forward" electronic transmission, and remote patient monitoring (RPM) are examples of such technologies. There are other potential applications of digital technology for patient management, such as monitoring, wearable technologies, online triage, online sources of health information, online booking of appointments, remote consultation, online access to health records, and the use of apps.

5. It enhances health service outcomes through increased accessibility and efficiency via reinforcing efforts to improve the quality of health service by providing clinical assistance, reducing geographic

boundaries, offering alternative communication devices, and enhancing patient results.

FOUR MAIN MODALITIES USED FOR TELEMEDICINE

1. **Interactive audio-video technology (live video):** Can conduct live video interaction between patient and physician.

2. **Store-and-forward technology:** Basic store-and-forward e-mail-based telemedicine technologies require little investment in hardware and software where network connectivity is accessible and allows for detailed interactions by allowing the transmission of imagery files as attachments, making it an effective solution for limited resource locations.

3. **Remote patient monitoring technology:** Remote patient monitoring (RPM) allows healthcare professionals to track patients' health information from distant locations, usually while the sick person is at their place of residence. RPM also can decrease the time a patient requires spending in the hospital, instead allowing them to convalesce under observation at their home. RPM is efficient for chronic conditions, such as heart disease, diabetes, and asthma.

4. **Mobile health technology:** This makes healthcare services more available, provides improved and rapid access, and is more affordable. The technology also provides easy ways for healthcare providers to check patient information, monitor outpatient health information, gather records when at a patient's bedside, educate and coach healthcare providers - especially, those working in remote and rural areas.

This technology supports pharmacists and diverse health care professionals to aid and evaluate patients' prescriptions for adherence, chronic care conditions, and isolated patient monitoring.

PART 2:
ORIGIN AND GLOBAL HISTORY OF TELEMEDICINE USAGE

According to several published articles, telemedicine originated in the middle of the 19th century and was mainly reported in the early 20th Century. It was more formally adopted between the late 1960s and early 1970s and used in the military and space industry workforces.[121-123] Additional published peer-reviewed research claims the first technological breakthroughs in telemedicine platforms came in the form of using television to promote consultations between professionals, general practitioners, and patients at a state psychiatric institution [124] However, the replacement of analog forms of connection with digital techniques, associated with a fast reduction in the cost of information and communication technologies, has stimulated wide involvement in the application of telemedicine among health-care providers and has enabled health care establishments to foresee and achieve greater economic measures in offering healthcare services to needy populations.[125, 126]

Current improvements and growing opportunities to use the latest information and communication technologies have been significant drivers of telemedicine over the previous decade, forming new opportunities for health care service and delivery.[127] These developments have led to the formation of a valuable drapery of telemedicine applications (e-mail, teleconsultations, and conferences via the Internet) and multimedia approaches (digital imagery and video) that everyone is now using daily.

PART 3:
COMPONENTS AND SYSTEMS NEEDED TO IMPLEMENT TELEMEDICINE

We can categorize telemedicine technologies into two significant types corresponding to the effectiveness of the data transferred and the synergy between the users: Store-and-forward or asynchronous and synchronous processes. Asynchronous describes the relationship between two or more events/objects that interact within the same system but do not occur at predetermined intervals and do not rely on each other's existence to act. In synchronous processes, however, the events/object or personal communication between recipients must occur at once and they can respond at their convenience.[128]

Store-and-forward, or asynchronous processes in telemedicine requires a network of pre-documented information among two or more people at various periods. In comparison, in real-time or synchronous processes the engaged persons need to be present for a prompt network of knowledge as with videoconferencing. In both synchronous and asynchronous telemedicine processes a transfer of significant data may be accomplished via a string of channels such as text, audio, video, or still images.

There are advantages and disadvantages to both processes of delivery.

Asynchronous is simple, practical, and applied for carrying limited amounts of data. Synchronous delivery is applied for sending larger quantities of data as it is economical and allows less overhead.[129]

Such applications will unquestionably advance the delivery of health services in Africa, the U.S. Virgin Islands, and Haiti by not only migrating health care delivery away from hospitals and clinics into homes, but further by linking health-care providers with specialists, referral hospitals, and healthcare institutions.

PART 4:
LITERATURE EVALUATION APPROACH

Literature evaluated for this book included existing scientific literature to define the prevailing state of telemedicine technologies in African countries, the USVI, and Haiti. Also, included in the evaluations were reviews that reported on telemedicine usage and interactions of healthcare providers, patient, stakeholders, and community's representative results, research and assessment procedures, educational outcomes, and cost-effective measurements. Scientific examinations and analysis and analytic editorials based on the benchmarks delineated below were also chosen and evaluated.

EVALUATION BENCHMARKS

Applicants: Included healthcare professionals, patients, and community populations using healthcare services provided through telemedicine platforms in African countries, the USVI, and Haiti.

Interventions: Comprised of studies exploring any incidence of telemedicine implementation related to the targeted areas identified within this book.

Results: Research findings were included if they analyzed telemedicine outcomes related to healthcare services, quality of healthcare, research, and education of healthcare providers.

Date: Publication of research editorials and articles: Editorials and articles deemed valid for review, consideration, and inclusion in the book were confined to research available from January 1980 to the present.

Language: Editorials and articles included those available in English only; however, other studies written in other languages were also consulted.

Research prohibition benchmarks: Rejected editorials and articles included those in which the primary aim of the telemedicine platform use was not related to public health improvement and access to quality healthcare services. The evaluation also rejected studies that centered on mobile phones and other wireless appliances.

Literature examination approach: The following research systems, databases, and online platforms were used to locate and identify articles within the timeline of January 1980 to the present:

- The Medical Literature Analysis and Retrieval System Online (MEDLINE)
- The WHO and CDC Database indexes including:
  - African Index Medicus (AIM)
  - Latin American and Caribbean Health Sciences (LILACS) produced by the Pan American Health Organization (PAHO) Institutional Memory Database
  - The WHO Library Database (WHOLIS) using the WHO Global Health Library platform (www.globalhealthlibrary.net)
  - The Telecare and Telemedicine Journal and e-Health.

The following search terms were used to focus on the scope of research for evaluation: telemedicine, telehealth, African countries, the U.S. Virgin Islands, and Haiti. The literature examination also included references from retrieved reports, articles, and unofficial reports.

Choice of studies: Retrieved data, editorials, and articles were assessed to uncover those to be merged in the assessment. However, retrieved data from editorials and articles established not to satisfy the criteria to include in the evaluation were rejected. Review outcomes included 350 articles. Based on the criteria delineated above, 50 of these were identified not significant and therefore omitted from the evaluation. The total sum of editorials and articles considered was over three hundred (300).

PART 5:
BENEFITS OF TELEMEDICINE TO IMPROVING ACCESS AND HEALTHCARE QUALITY

As of today, most of the populations in the USVI, Haiti, and a substantial number of African nations, according to published sources, including the World Health Organization and World Bank observatory data, have an average life expectancy of below 70 years, compared to those in developed countries such as Hong Kong - 84.3, and the United States of America - 76 years. Although the USA has a lower life expectancy than most other developed countries, at 76 years, this is still higher than most African nations, USVI, and Haiti.[130-131] People living in rural and remote localities are more expected than urban inhabitants to have increased mortality due to leading diseases such as heart disease, cancer, unintentional injury, chronic lower respiratory disease, and stroke. Therefore, a more patient-centered care approach should substitute the conventional standard of irregular and public health-based care, in which patients are linked to their primary doctors. The high mortality should, of necessity motivate the initiation and implementation of referendums to change and improve the success of the disrupted health care system and allow innovations in technology, such as the integration and implementation of telemedicine services.

There is substantial evidence to support the effective and efficient performance of telemedicine services and technologies. Published data and articles have disclosed that telemedicine services encourage constancy of healthcare service, reduces the expense of care, and enhances people with self-reliance, assistance, and comprehensive medical results. For instance, evidence published in a 2019 study related to the remote management of heart failure patients established that telemonitoring decreased death and heart failure associated with hospital care.[132-133]

Telemedicine can also help discover and avoid treatment-associated inaccuracies between hospital or clinic consultations, especially in distant localities. As one instance demonstrated in published reports that prescription errors can be decreased by telemedicine use.[134-135] Doctor-correlated medication errors were also revealed to be reduced in people who received telemedicine consultations in comparison to those who received in-person consultations. [136, 137] And an additional study reports comparable decreases in prescription mistakes when Telepharmacy is used.[138]

Incorporating and implementing telemedicine technology in the current disrupted healthcare systems can reduce obstacles to care for people living distant from healthcare specialists or who have transportation and mobility problems. The technology platforms are an effective approach to providing rapid care in urgent situations such as stroke. Further better monitoring, through telemedicine can improve patients' quality of life, shorten hospital admissions, and prevent losses from chronic diseases.

In summation, supporting the implementation of telemedicine services across African countries, the USVI, and Haiti to provide vulnerable populations with better access to chronic disease prevention and management programs and specialist care, such as (stroke care and cardiac recovery, diabetes care and prevention programs, vision care for individuals with diabetes, tobacco cessation, and epilepsy management) is a significant motivation to proceed forward with this approach. [139]

As mentioned already, the delivery of health services, especially in rural and remote regions, is disrupted by reduced funding and other resource limitations, such as continuous decreases in infrastructure funding support for health facilities in these areas.

Targeted consideration of population healthcare delivery needs in rural and remote areas is vital and speaks to the WHO idea of 'Health for All' articulated in the Declaration of Alma Ata in 1978: "…that health is a state of complete physical, mental and social wellbeing and not the absence of disease or infirmity; that health is a fundamental human right; and that the attainment of the highest possible level of health is a most important worldwide social goal". Further, the Declaration of Alma Ata continues to state that: "Governments have a responsibility for the health of their people which can be fulfilled only by the provision of adequate health and social measures. Bringing health care as close as possible to where people live and work and should constitute the first level of a continuing health care process." [140-142]

The incorporation of telemedicine technology into healthcare systems worldwide, but especially in poorer and developing nations, could serve to fulfill the mandate of the Declaration of Alma Ata by making access to a higher level of health care accessible to all. It is more than possible that the implementation of this technology could take the delivery of medical care to an entirely new level resulting in far more equitable and affordable services. *The Health for All Rural People: The Durban Declaration,* held in Durban, South Africa in 1997, outlined "a series of principles which should be followed by a Call for Action renewing the 'Health for All' initiatives and calling on the

WHO, the UNICEF, development banks such as the World Bank and other regional development banks, and national governments to address the historical inequities facing rural and disadvantaged communities. The Declaration also recommended that targets be set in stages until the year 2020 to reduce all aspects of global poverty, social, cultural, economic, education, nutritional, and health disparities. [143]

- Beside the benefits listed above, the following sections outline other advantages which have been shown to improve access to quality health services and decrease significant health inequity faced by the population.
- Telemedicine can assist doctor-patient examinations in the long-term, as it offers healthcare providers possibilities for case-based education that can be used in the treatment of patients. [144, 145] Incorporation of technical resources also gives health-care providers the chance to gain technological expertise transferrable to other situations. [146]
- Linking several distant locations via telemedicine technologies may be a beneficial approach providing access to quality healthcare service to these areas, when measured with the choice of actually erecting facilities and recruiting healthcare providers, especially healthcare specialists. [147] There is opportunity to utilize both hard structures and telemedicine technology together as buildings have tremendous capacity and appropriateness in the aspect of surges and disasters, while telecommunications can offer a channel between emergency room healthcare providers and colleagues at distant or disaster locations.
- Additional indirect potential telemedicine can provide African countries, the USVI, and Haiti the readiness to harmonize and gather patient information. Telemedicine platforms can assist epidemiological surveying by aiding in detecting and mapping issues (such as outbreak)

and showing progression. [148] This type of focused communication regarding infectious outbreak / disease progression allows for better oversight and enables support to design and assemble response units. [149] Also, certain telemedicine systems can enhance information management via network databanks and electronic recording processes. This can improve more managed care while enabling the possibility for more patient follow-up and assessment.

- Improvement in technology including the development of telemedicine services in African countries, the USVI, and Haiti and widespread use of the technology will encourage the cost of Information Communication Technologies (ICTs) to fall, thus making the overall cost of implementation and maintenance of the services and technology less burdensome to governments and healthcare systems. [150, 151] Other related services will also benefit from the incorporation of telemedicine technologies, including: improving computing speeds, and greater possibilities for high-speed capacity, and the decrease in rates for digital storage capacity. [152] Low bandwidth, internet-based telemedicine platforms such as (store and forward, and e-mail-based consultations) also have cost-effective technology that can be used to examine, in advance, patients residing in isolated regions. [153] Through improving the data transmission technology structure and enhancing better communication facilities, telemedicine services can similarly add to the better management of insufficient resources and daily activities in African countries, the USVI, and Haiti. [154]
- Basic store-and-forward e-mail-based telemedicine technologies have minor investment requirements in hardware and software where network connectivity is accessible and allows for detailed interactions by fostering the transmission of imagery files as attachments,

making it an effective solution for limited resource locations. [155, 156] The growing expansion of Internet-based teleconferencing, mainly via costless software, raises the availability and portability of this format and counters the need for costly video teleconferencing equipment that may have limited accessibility. [157]

TELEMEDICINE CLOSES THE GAP IN SPECIALTY REFERRALS

Substantial obstacles to promptly accessing specialty care services are endured by the poor and rural populations of African countries, the USVI, and Haiti. These include a broken healthcare system, lack of universal health insurance, a significant shortage of specialists, and frequent absence of networking among primary care providers and specialists.

Enhancing the use of existing specialty resources through telemedicine platforms will save people time, effort, and concern. It will also be cost-effective for chronic disease services and contribute to decreasing the gap in specialty referrals. Telemedicine platforms can provide connectivity between the primary healthcare provider and selected specialists to exchange patients' medical histories and decide the best treatment pathway.

TELEMEDICINE AIMS TO AVOID UNNECESSARY EMERGENCY ROOM VISITS

Emergency rooms in African countries, the USVI, and Haiti are always congested, costly, and can be frightening places to go; telemedicine services can prevent needless ambulance trips and unnecessary burdening of emergency room services and resources.

Using telemedicine services through a simple click with a smartphone, computer, or tablet, could save a life, time, and financial burdening by allowing patients and/or family members, from the comfort of their homes, to communicate virtually with doctors or nurses for proper follow-up medication and treatments.

Integrating, and implementing telemedicine platforms into the healthcare system will help emergency rooms' healthcare providers focus more on injuries and medical conditions that warrant emergency room services. This will reduce the use of emergency rooms as non-emergency care centers whose role is to focus on minor injuries and infections that demand minimal physical examination along with providing resources, services, and educational material so patients achieve better health.

Such beneficial approaches will decrease emergency medical transportation services and be a cost-effective saving for poor people living in urban, rural, and remote areas, along with allowing healthcare providers to become more proactive instead of reactive.

HEALTHCARE PROVIDERS BENEFIT FROM TELEMEDICINE PLATFORMS

For healthcare providers, telemedicine can be a major boost to their practice. Used in conjunction with other advanced medical technology, telemedicine has the propensity to increase the profit margin for providers, contribute to improving workflow, save and enhance return on investment, and lessen provider burnout. Telemedicine offers complete satisfaction to both patients and physicians and can increase revenue streams. Enhanced financial earnings can serve as a motivating factor to instill the services, but also to improve provider retention. Those health professionals considering departing the medical field due to factors related to diminished financial benefits and decreasing job contentment may find the ease of telemedicine and its accompanying increased financial benefits sufficient to remain. These factors, coupled with improved patient care via the technology, may be strong motivational factors leading to provider satisfaction, and thereby, retention. Work-life balance for healthcare practitioners and providers may also benefit from telemedicine as the platform allows for work and/or consultation outside conventional work hours, thus allowing providers to set hours that suit them and their patients' lifestyles.

As telemedicine platforms become more common, and the cost becomes less prohibitive, more ways to increase revenue streams via the medium may become apparent as more providers employ the technology.

REMOTE AND RURAL COMMUNITIES' BENEFIT FROM TELEMEDICINE'S ACCESSIBILITY

Remote and rural communities, segregated by geography, are a significant characteristic of much of the African and Caribbean countryside. For the past decades, access to quality healthcare services has been problematic for populations residing in such areas. Although, some basic health care services are available, people encounter a host of obstacles in efforts to get much needed care.

One of the foremost obstacles to accessibility is distance. In many African nations especially, distances to local health clinics are well out of the reach of everyday persons, and public transportation is non-existent, causing persons in need to walk miles before they can access care.

The lack of effective public or private transportation to fulfill medical appointments, especially for senior citizens and the disabled remains a constant obstacle compared to those who live in urban localities.

Another factor affecting accessibility is cost. Without national health insurance programs, most citizens must pay for health care out of pocket, and services are expensive. In addition, for those who are employed, taking time off work for medical reasons, means doing so without pay – something few can afford on low wage jobs. The stress of illness coupled with lack of access compounds morbidity in the aged, the disabled, and those residing in remote or rural areas.

In many of these areas the preeminent healthcare provider is a primary care doctor, and if these are not available, or inaccessible due to lack of transportation or funds, many simply forego the care they need resulting in a significant increase in health disparities or deaths within the communities.

Telemedicine is perceived as a valued answer to this challenging situation wherein lack of accessibility and cost are driving components of the inequity. Through telemedicine platforms, the need for travel is negated, thus remote and rural populations can receive specialists' diagnosis and treatment time while remaining in their home or community hospitals. It can also contribute to reduced mortality, support people with mobility limitations, decrease extended stay in health institutions, reduce evaluation time for mental health practitioners, and avert unneeded, burdensome costs for travel.

Telemedicine will also promote partnership and a work environment of mutual learning among healthcare providers, and diminish the hierarchy perceived between rural health-care providers and urban specialists, which will reduce the grasp of discrimination expressed by many healthcare providers practicing in provincial and poor communities.

Overall, the telemedicine platform constitutes a significant opportunity from both a clinical and financial viewpoint since it will not only empower healthcare providers to broaden best practices, but also allow people living in distant and neglected communities to have reliable access to high-quality health services irrespective of location, and that is also cost saving for poor people.

PART 6:
THE ROLE OF TELEMEDICINE IN IMPROVING MEDICAL EDUCATION OR CONTINUING EDUCATION FOR PROVIDERS

As telemedicine has become an essential part of healthcare delivery systems around the world, its inclusion in the training of healthcare providers, including teachers and students, has likewise become needed and significant. Therefore, to further leverage these technologies, governments must ensure healthcare providers practice their use as well. Up to now, the utilization of telemedicine platforms and technology for medical and continuing education of healthcare providers has been restricted to just a few study settings, instead of being an important element of the medical and continuing education curriculum.

It is imperative to understand the international framework into which the telemedicine medical and continuing education in African countries, the USVI, and Haiti occurs.

Parallel with developed countries such as Australia, France, and the United States, to name just a few, which have relied heavily on telemedicine services because of geographic boundaries and recent COVID-19 outbreak, African countries, the USVI, and Haiti still have much progress to achieve.[158, 159]

During the COVID-19 pandemic ailing persons were being encouraged to stay at home even if presenting with minor symptoms. To help with the provision and availability of medical care to augment overburdened hospitals the World Health Organization (WHO) and federal health agencies including the Food and Drug Administration (FDA) and Centers for Disease Control and Prevention (CDC) made telemedicine platforms less challenging for both patients and healthcare providers.[160-161]

The importance of telemedicine training in medical and continuing education has been expressed by healthcare providers promoting and encouraging the implementation of telemedicine curricula by all institutions, including medical schools, throughout African countries, the USVI, and Haiti. While formulating any new medical education program can appear frightening, it is believed that telemedicine education can be integrated into existing curriculums. This integration is essential for the long-term implementation and progress of telemedicine in these countries. Emerging efforts that expose healthcare providers to the use of telemedicine have been successful in a few African and developing countries.

As telemedicine services rise and evermore significant technology is developed, governments must collaborate with governing bodies, including healthcare provider associations, to improve compensation and remove accrediting roadblocks, thereby helping to ensure healthcare providers perceive telemedicine platforms as essential components of their work environment and productivity. This can only be achieved by eliminating traditional practice biases and preparing healthcare providers to deliver care across traditional and non-traditional platforms. To accomplish this, telemedicine medical and continuing education programs must pursue increased exposure in concert with knowledge of multifaceted governmental, socioeconomic, and cultural principles involved. This is significant considering the fast pace of technological modernization. Healthcare providers must not only be educated to practice medicine using telemedicine platforms but do so in an evidence-based approach.[162]

Transparency in the efforts of African countries, the USVI, and Haiti to integrate telemedicine training into their curricula and discourse involving best practices needs to be promoted. Therefore, formal training is the best method for teaching healthcare providers how to approach the challenges and opportunities inherent in telemedicine practice.

By definition "formal training occurs in a structured environment such as a training or educational institution or on the job. They design it as education in terms of time, objectives, and resources. Sergiy Movchan, an expert in e-learning, defines formal learning as: "intentional learning from the learner's perspective, leading to degrees and certifications. Formal learning is a structured model that presents a rigid curriculum, corresponding to laws and norms. It is rather presentational education." [163] Such formal learning generally takes place in structured environments such as schools; however, on the job training is also formal training. On the other hand, "informal learning is that which is provided through life experiences, through learning projects, peer groups, family, media, and other venues outside traditional formalized learning environments (schools, universities, business programs, etc.).[164]

Simply put, the difference between formal and informal training refers to what is studied with determination and what is learned by experience on the job or by accident. Today's healthcare providers are a breed of digital natives', e.g., individuals raised with digital technology as a normal part of their surroundings and are therefore comfortable processing information in a computerized system.

Healthcare providers' essential satisfaction with technology must be fostered through organized training. Without this, they will be unable to benefit from modern innovations in current and developing telemedicine technologies. The creation and implementation of a formal training program will allow providers to correlate and contrast telemedicine programs with conventional medical practice strategies, recognize when to use it, and gain knowledge on best practices.

The successfulness of this approach requires the structure of programs be meaningful and comprehensive. Thus, collaborative endeavors between African countries, within the USVI, and throughout the Haitian government are needed. Further, to ensure effectiveness in telemedical care services, these governments must train healthcare providers to engage in telemedicine programs with the exact same dexterity they show in delivering conventional care.

TELEMEDICINE SERVICES IN A HEALTHCARE CONTEXT

Millions in African countries, Haiti, and thousands in the USVI live in urban and rural areas. For these people, affordable and accessible quality health care at the local level is scarce. Geographic isolation combined with population densities makes the provision of sustainable local health care in rural areas a challenge. Also, insufficient, and inadequate local resources combined with difficulties in recruiting and retaining physicians further complicates local access to quality health care.

As a result, these populations are forced to travel interminable distances to get medical treatment at considerable time and expense not only for the patient, but also for friends and family. Those unable to bear the expense may forgo treatment altogether, risking a health care crisis. Telemedicine platforms are an important solution to the challenges of health care access in rural areas.

It can connect rural and remote patients with general physicians and medical specialists located outside the patients' communities.

As the demand for robust healthcare systems has increased throughout African countries, the USVI, and Haiti, the promising potential of telemedicine services will reinforce the message that there is an across the board need to enhance the quality of healthcare systems through improving convenience and effectiveness by decreasing the necessity to travel, offering medical assistance, presenting multiple communication mechanisms, and enhancing people's welfare.

The implementation of telemedicine as a regular and necessary component of overall medical care can be an effective approach for complementing the current disrupted health care services. It can also draw attention to and place emphasis on attempts to curb expenditures and enhance the delivery of care to all sectors of the population.

It is in this direction that resolution WHA58.28 was drafted by the member nations of the 2005 World Health Assembly. The resoluion stated that the member nations would agree to establish long term sustainable eHealth strategies, provide needed telecommunications infrastructure, and create effective national centers.[165, 166] While telemedicine platforms will not resolve all the health difficulties confronting these countries, it can be viewed as one of the contemporary technologies with the ability to leverage and offer healthcare services where distance is a serious issue.

As the worldwide Web has developed into an integral part of present-time survival with it uses in business, education, politics, entertainment, and healthcare, there are those who believe that telemedicine, through a Web-based disease management system, can also be seen as an answer to supporting people with chronic diseases in the self-care and management of their illnesses.[167]

Web-based disease management programs will invite people to embrace better accountability for their care, assist healthcare professionals in giving medical care or attention to individuals before illness occurs, offer the most cost-effective services, expand limited healthcare resources, improve continuity of care, improve access to health services, and expand the efficiency and quality of medical records. [168] Implementing this technology covers a wide scope, including online databases and devices to provide quality of health care, computer-assisted analysis, efficient medication data and automated drug filling, and improved accessibility of information.

Included in the healthcare provisions for most chronic diseases is the need to contain immediate and future associated costs. Implicit within this approach is the building of sound physician-patient relationship with the onus of accountability upon the patient to make lifestyle changes and adhere to medication protocols.

Diabetes and other avoidable chronic illnesses are among those having a critical need to reduce healthcare expenditures through lifestyle improvements and effective care strategies. This implies that people suffering from chronic diseases have the ability to control illness onset and progression by following the advice of healthcare providers and maintaining established care routines which aid in reducing potential problems which add to the cost and expense of care. Diabetes is a prime example because without proper care and maintenance it can lead to other life-threatening diseases and conditions such as neuropathy – resulting in amputation, glaucoma and blindness, increased risk of heart disease and stroke, all of which increase the costs of the disease.

Further, through telemedicine technology, healthcare providers would be able to treat and supervise many more people than typical care practices could tolerate. This expansion of the patient base improves access to many associated levels of health services and specialists to carry out better curative objectives, in patient's homes instead of in hospitals, clinic, and nursing home care settings. [169, 170]

Using smart surveillance cameras and diagnostic software through telemedicine technology would also enable healthcare providers to remotely check upon the health status of the elderly population and inform their caregivers of developments, inactivity, falls, or death.

This form of telemedicine care can decrease expenses, allow the elderly to remain in their places of residence longer, and assist healthcare providers (specialists) in personalizing medication according to the individual's preferences and convenience of care. The availability of such point of care services are urgent as it is primarily the aging populations of African countries, the USVI, and Haiti who are living longer without substantial simultaneous improvements in funding supports for healthcare services and infrastructure.

The elderly populations of African nations are projected to reach 67 million by 2025 and 163 million by 2050. It is further anticipated that by 2025, individuals 65 years or older will represent 22% of the USVI population, and some 800,000 Haitians over 60 currently live-in extreme poverty.[171-175] Therefore, healthcare services and infrastructure will continue to cope with significant financial challenges as the ratio of the population needing additional health services will increase.

Using telemedicine platforms can assist individuals requiring care and treatment for an injury, as via the technology physicians and specialists can provide information, view the injury, the patient can upload and share pictures of the injury, and a diagnosis and treatment regimen or referral for further care and services can all be provided.

As of today, the governments of the nations addressed in this work have not initiated minimal effort and engagement to promote and enhance telemedicine services. It has been shown that a lack of development of telemedicine services, most times, discourages health care providers and the population from attempting to use it.

Therefore, this book attempts to explore the impediments to telemedicine implementation from previous and existing experiences in a few African countries, USVI, and Haiti. Although various factors could affect the adoption and use of telemedicine services, this book shows that the use of this technology platform could contribute to decreasing barriers to providing access to quality health services to the population at large.

Using and improving existing internet-based connections such as e-mail, medical web portals, and top speed-capacity to carry out health-care services and offer teleconsultations are encouraging factors that can help move this effort forward.

Implementing telemedicine services also requires re-igniting and improving the collaborative efforts of all the healthcare actors, stakeholders, and enhancing awareness and skills training for medical and professional staff in other disciplines to embrace this technology.

As telemedicine spans a continuum of technologies that could offer different approaches in providing safe management and continual care for millions, doctors, nurses, and social workers who embody the essential group of healthcare providers, must undergo multicourse training that recognizes and reflects the uniqueness of technology-mediated services.

The teaching offered must be thorough and developed in a telemedicine work context. Ensuring an experienced and resource capable and equipped healthcare workforce for urban, rural, and remote regions is important and necessary to promoting health of the population. The training should place emphasis on outlining the delivery of telemedicine interventions that are mediated through technology. It should also address legal and ethical concerns and assist healthcare providers in evaluating when such services are convenient for individuals, especially those who are living in remote and rural areas as there can be connectivity issues or limitations in such areas.

Implementing and incorporating telemedicine technology platforms also has an administrative component wherein there is a demand for formal policies, regulations, and strategies to regulate health service delivery and assess quality of care. Consequently, healthcare providers should be trained in and gain the skills fundamental to handling these responsibilities. The multicourse must also cover practice in group-based interventions that will delve into matters such as developing delivery healthcare systems that can enhance patient involvement, retention, and increase health services results. Further, healthcare providers could learn how to interact with their associates, share meaningful exchanges, and draw on telemedicine work expertise as they confront issues, especially those working in remote communities.

One of the foremost challenges facing the governments of African countries, the USVI, and Haiti is consideration of the social, political, and economic consequences of telemedicine platforms and the need to create pathways to expand their use and processes to all the population, especially neglected people living in rural and remote areas.

CHAPTER THREE:
BRINGING TELEMEDICINE TO AFRICA, HAITI, AND THE USVI

PART 1:
TELEMEDICINE PILOT PROJECTS IN AFRICA, HAITI, AND THE USVI

Among the different elements that structure the variety of healthcare services provided via the Internet, telemedicine services, defined "as the use of telecommunication and information technology to provide and improve access to medical services that would not be available in distant rural communities," has garnered the utmost attention.[176, 177] Although there are a lot of available articles showing the possible use of telemedicine services in many African countries, the U.S. Virgin Islands, and Haiti, our field observation found there are few significant, ongoing initiatives that carry out telemedicine services in the African continent, the USVI, and Haiti. However, these few determined attempts continue to be undermined, secluded, and sometimes unproductive from the principal aims.

While it might be problematic to define with certainty a particular moment when telemedicine services were introduced into these areas, several published and unpublished reviews show, that a few countries - South Africa, Ghana, Nigeria, Uganda, and Kenya - embraced the use of partial telemedicine services into their public health industries several years ago. Reports show that these countries were moving in the direction that could improve and offer substantial conditions and accessible healthcare benefits to their entire populations.[178-181]

Several other African nations - Botswana, Burundi, Cote de Ivoire, Djibouti, Egypt, Eritrea, Libya, Malawi, Mozambique, Somalia, and Zambia - were involved in telemedicine pilot projects such as the fundamental of modern telemedicine for Africa (FOMTA), the Pan-African e-network project (PANP) and the Reseau en Afrique Francophone pour la Telemedicine (RAFT).[182, 183]

Meanwhile, the countries of Mali, Sudan, Rwanda, and Burkina Faso were promoting the use of telemedicine technology to provide better approaches to enhanced health care services, reduce prices, and reduce the critical shortage of physicians across several disciplines. However, because of nationwide economic restrictions, Burkina Faso suspended its exploratory use of telemedicine services.[184-189]

The USDA Rural Development Peer Report in March 2018 revealed that the U.S. Virgin Islands gained its first experience with telemedicine technologies through distance learning projects established in 2009 on St. John at the Myrah Keating Clinic. USDA provided the technology through cooperation with the Cleveland Clinic in Weston, Florida; however, the project ended February 21, 2013 due to a shortage of adequate funding. In its last year, there were 90 appointments to the clinic that were made using telemedicine platforms. Thus, the project experience was limited. [190]

The distrust constantly displayed by those using the current healthcare system alongside continual disparities in access to quality care between and within the islands of the USVI, remains an interesting motivation for integrating these technology platforms. Also, the platform can expand services as a single clinician can reach more patients using the technology, thus addressing, and reducing physician shortages.

Haiti has not produced effective data about past practices using telemedicine programs, but the western hemisphere's poorest country is not unfamiliar with the technology's platforms, especially after the 7.0-magnitude earthquake in January 2010 that killed 300,000 individuals. Prior to the earthquake, implementing telemedicine was not regarded as a priority because conflict, political uncertainty, and environmental deterioration decimated the country. [191]

The catastrophic earthquake of 2010 brought with it the opportunity for implementing telemedicine platforms to meet the needs of so many injured across the island and to augment the existing but scarce health service infrastructure. The disaster strengthened the advancement of telemedicine services which were provided through a pilot project of the University of Miami. The project brought telemedicine into the country's rural interior. Telemedicine and alternative communications technology, mobile tech, were exploited to support Haitian doctors in their efforts to perform in what was left behind as public health facilities.[192] The University of Miami telemedicine project was a tremendous experience. The enthusiasm of many private healthcare providers and international non-profit institutions for incorporating telemedicine services within Haiti's fractured healthcare organizations has been unparalleled.

Although there are an absence of data illustrating any current practice of telemedicine services in Haiti, our field examination, discovered that a few initiatives such as Telemedicine Coordination for Haiti Relief through the American Telemedicine Association (ATA) and iCONS in Medicine, formed Haiti SA, Telemedicine at Hospital Sacre Coeur initiative, and Center of Telemedicine Polyclinic Turgeau are involved in providing segmented telemedicine services to the population.[193-195]

These telemedicine providers have been complementing a fragmented health structure. It will be most consistent if the technology is fully implemented, operative, and sustainable throughout the country so it can enhance access to quality healthcare service for all of Haiti's impoverished people.

Haiti's political situation has improved in recent years, however, civil chaos, such as regular protests and labor force strikes, political violence, frequent business disruption, and land assaults by unlawful tenants in both urban and rural areas, have continued to be major issues for the island nation. Prevalent corruption also remains an obstacle, and political rallies, along with periodic confrontations, occur often in the capital city of Port-au-Prince. [196, 197] Overall, the country continues to experience unrest, high unemployment, disruption of services, disease outbreaks, and man-made and natural disasters, all of which leave its populous beaten into lives of misery constantly striving for survival. All these conditions dramatically impact access and availability of health care services.

Leaning on the expertise of developed countries, especially those involved and advanced in the ongoing processes of development, implementation, and maintenance of telemedicine systems, is important for these countries as they consider the technology for more full-time use. Focusing on best practices and lessons learned from other more experienced nations will help stakeholders, healthcare providers, and community populations with choosing the right infrastructure and technology (broadband and vetting equipment capacity). Looking to this wide array of readily available knowledge can also prove helpful in locating the right (or best) vendor(s) and improving any existing telemedicine policies, regulatory barriers, and billing guidance for reimbursement.

As of today, the healthcare systems in many African countries, and Haiti are worsening despite significant efforts from unprecedented levels of funding to improve access to suitable, quality health service delivery of the population at large.

The World Health Organization Regional Office for Africa, 2013 report, confirms that despite slight development improvement in many countries, the member states of the WHO African Region are still far from completing their health funding targets to achieve the Abuja proposal of allotting 15% of government resources to health and decreasing the out-of-pocket expenses in all health spending. [198]

The U. S. Virgin Islands has not fared much better than some African nations in its efforts to establish and maintain a fully functioning healthcare system. Prior to hurricanes Irma and Maria, the territory funded its public health services through Wall Street financing that was manifested through the purchase of triple tax-exempt bonds, by investors. By 2017, the island territory was indebted to its creditors for more than $2 billion dollars. The health system, along with other public services, has continued to suffer enduring more shortages and insufficiencies since the hurricanes.[199]

Despite the efforts of multiple lenders – from other governments and private non-governmental organizations – the financial obligations to improve public health systems in African countries, the USVI, and Haiti (WHO, 2003) remain stalled. Along with an unprecedented level of funding received from mainly international donations, the health of the overall populations, especially those living in poor and sidelined communities, remains at risk and is still afflicted by diseases that are preventable and curable. [200, 201] Access, equity, quality, and cost-effectiveness are yet considerable core challenges for the population.

In light of these issues the governments of African nations, the USVI, and Haiti should strengthen the capacity of healthcare services by improving the health infrastructure, reducing the healthcare provider shortage, implement universal health coverage, and incorporate telemedicine technologies into the healthcare system to leverage efforts and possibilities to build a stronger health system.

Telemedicine platforms involving computers, internet, and cell phones, to refer to just a few, are revolutionizing how people relate not only with their physicians but also with each other to exchange information and enhance their lives. Telemedicine technology has considerable potential to help address the contemporary health problems of these areas. Expanding the spectrum of health interventions through integrating telemedicine platforms will contribute to improvement and respond to the needs of underprivileged populations regarding access to quality health systems and delivery capability.

PART 2:
IMPLEMENTING TELEMEDICINE TODAY

As of now, telemedicine platforms hold considerable promise for decreasing the inconsistency of diagnoses, along with enhancing the delivery of health care services by improving access, excellence, effectiveness, and cost-efficiency.

There are indications that the use of telemedicine platforms and services may result in improved socioeconomic advantages to the population, healthcare providers, and the healthcare system, as well as improving patient-doctor conversation and fostering partnership between distant healthcare providers and urban healthcare workers (doctors).[202] Telemedicine services may encourage specialists to remain in rural practices through reinforcement of professional assistance and prospects for pursuing professional growth. [203]

Field assessments conducted by ICAN, coupled with several published reviews, conclude that the technology allows healthcare providers the opportunity to share information through video conferencing and secure sharing of patient data and records with other doctors, thereby improving the results of patient treatments.[204-207] Thus, the ability of this technology will be substantial in African countries, USVI, and Haiti, where not only the shortage of physicians is growing each year, but also the quality of current public health structures creates difficulties that impede the ability to provide better health services to the population. Therefore, offering these populations better ways to access quality health care services through telemedicine platforms will help reach unmet demands and, in the long term, establish the country's health system. However, despite its enormous potential, technological and financial barriers such as lack of expansive broadband service, transmitting video, audio, and imaging via emerging telecommunications infrastructure restrict its widespread implementation.

In the aforementioned countries, telemedicine has not been widely adopted and used to offer access to quality healthcare services. Presently, just a few attempted initiatives have proven successful in upholding themselves after primary funding was completed. Our assessments, combined with those referenced in published articles, revealed several challenges leading to diminished capacity and reduced longevity with the comprehensive implementation of several telemedicine service projects.

There are some – politicians, healthcare providers, and citizens – who oppose implementing service designs that deviate from customary operations and practices; while others resist because more knowledge is needed to fully avail themselves of the benefits and uses of telemedicine services. Additional challenges included linguistic and cultural disparities between patients, especially those residing in underserved communities, and among healthcare providers.[208-211]

Another factor in the resistance to telemedicine services is the persistent lack of comprehensive and multidimensional improvement for better performance management. This is an essential point as performance management provides initiatives for improvement that can help gather, analyze, and communicate information about the cost-effectiveness of the practice of telemedicine services. Performance improvement also targets licensing and credentialing, data security and privacy, informed consent, peer review, and tailored performance improvement initiatives.[212] Such comprehensive and multidimensional performance improvement efforts are the heart of quality management and are critical to the justification of telemedicine.

Another serious challenge is the absence of a suitable, cost-effective health insurance market framework to reimburse healthcare providers for telemedicine services.

The Health insurance market is attracting more consideration as an alternative health funding system for enhancing access to quality health care and protecting the population against high out-of-pocket expenses. The World Health Organization (WHO) views health insurance as "a promising means for achieving universal health care coverage." Comprehensive health coverage aims to offer everyone, especially the impoverished, access to quality health services at a fair cost.[213, 214]

While Africa, the USVI and Haiti have incorporated Universal Health Coverage (UHC) as a goal in their national health strategies, progress in translating these promises into extended domestic resources for health, efficiency development support, fair and quality health services, and improved financial protection has been slow.

Health insurance in these countries represents "a tale of two cities": the very wealthy can take advantage of private insurance with top-tier doctors and hospitals while the extremely poor lack quality options. Many families, especially disadvantaged populations, depend on overcrowded state-run medical facilities with extended wait times and poor quality of care, or must pay out of pocket for health services. With disadvantaged populations paying over the counter, the health crisis has been causing severe financial hardship for families

Although health insurance is a multifaceted product, it is challenging to find a balance between public health goals and financial sustainability. However, defining the scope of treatment, the scale of treatment costs, the methods of reimbursement, and enhancing the quality of care and expanding distribution channels can improve the health coverage of the population.

These countries should provide access to affordable quality health services. More and improved Universal Health Coverage would transform health care in these countries.

Telemedicine has been rejected by some health care providers because of the inability of a fragile and vulnerable infrastructure ill-suited to support the rapid integration of telemedicine programs into their practices. Concerns have been expressed about depending on telemedicine infrastructures that are not effective, subject to unstable internet connectivity, and an unwillingness to properly learn how to use the equipment.

Effective integration of telemedicine programs requires sturdy platforms to facilitate video and audio communication and adoption of new billing codes. There is some concern about possible technology break down or disconnection during virtual consultations which can lead patients to follow the wrong treatment regimen. Also, the lack of understanding of how the consumer electronics market works and how it will provide physicians with the tools they need are all variables contributing to providers' reluctance to use telemedicine platforms.

Regulatory issues are another considerable drawback to telemedicine approval, including the absence of a worldwide lawful framework to empower healthcare providers to provide services from distant administrations and countries. A deficiency in guidelines that regulate confidentiality, data exchange, storage and sharing among health providers and jurisdictions, healthcare provider authentication related to e-mail submissions, and medical accountability for health providers eager to provide telemedicine technologies – all are additional issues.

The technological platforms present significant challenges because the techniques being used are multidimensional, and along with hardware equipment these remain a significant concern for users without professional competence. Although there are obstacles to successful telemedicine implementation, the benefits this technology holds for the healthcare industry are well worth the time and effort.

EXTERNAL IMPEDIMENTS TO ACHIEVING IMPROVED HEALTH CARE SYSTEMS

❖ *Corruption*

Corruption in the management of healthcare systems is recognized as a worldwide issue; however, in African countries, the USVI, and Haiti, this remains a primary contributing factor, according to the yearly Corruption Watch and transparency reports. The reports assert that corruption occurs foremost in the appearance of unusual expenditures, financial malpractice, embezzlement, unlawful distribution of patient data to third-party companies, cheating, and favoritism, to name a few, leading to medical services not being provided and healthcare providers and workers, occasionally not being paid. [215-217]

As of today, the singularity and difficulty with which public and private healthcare systems are structured and how this is related to and affects management effectiveness, increases vulnerability and susceptibility to corruption. The consequence is an unparalleled disparity in the affordability and quality of healthcare services. Continual misuse of public healthcare resources and frequent acceptance of bribes and irregular payments in return for favorable services are seriously compromising the quality of healthcare services.

Motivated by greed, people in charge of healthcare systems have been diverting critical resources away from the population in demand, causing insufficient resources, inferior quality of care, and deteriorating health results and outcomes. While preventing corruption in the healthcare industry looms as a multifaceted and problematic chore, implementing effective mechanisms, including effective auditing and liability, which should not simply reveal corruption but also condemn such actions to proper punishments, must be enforced. It is important to emphasize that such approaches will only succeed if they are unambiguous, transparent, and are accompanied by anti-corruption policies and procedures enforced with stringent measures and accountability standards.

Current laws and policies appear insufficient, therefore, a firm commitment from governments and policymakers to recognize and improve regulatory actions against corruption activities demand to be enhanced. Practical, improved strategies, and regulatory policies to recognize and identify corruption and punish it are significant approaches to promote and would serve to create an environment of deterrence. Further, governments should ensure that corruption in the healthcare industry does not affect the confidence of dedicated health care workers who are committed to providing the population with access to quality healthcare services.

❖ *Healthcare Provider Engagement*

Healthcare provider engagement remains a significant barrier to implementing telemedicine platforms. As of today, some medical professionals view telemedicine technologies as a potential competitor of their practices instead of as a means by which more patients may access medical services. One way to address the issue is to remind healthcare providers that telemedicine technology is a viable means of bringing medical care back to communities and into individual homes, especially, people residing in rural and underserved areas.

Adopting telemedicine technology will make medical practices more competitive and has the propensity to increase profits through the addition of more patients on-line as well as enhancing reimbursement opportunities from government, private insurance, and third-party payers. Further, it is advantageous for providers not to view telemedicine services as a competitor's benefit, but rather as a competitive edge for medical practices, and a means of preserving and enhancing doctor-patient confidentiality and relationships.

Beyond these suggestions, they must structure a partnership between governments and healthcare providers to ensure accuracy, security, safety, and appropriateness for exchanging sensitive data, especially when the communication is not synchronous. In conclusion, telemedicine will ease healthcare services and may have a major part in healthcare's future industry.

❖ *Physician Licensing*

Telemedicine services can facilitate a country's ability to conduct nationwide consultations, which will improve health care providers' ability to assist more people with health needs. The countries focused upon herein, are embracing telemedicine platforms by encouraging their use and advising health care providers to incorporate them into their practices. However, they have made little progress in removing medical licensing barriers that keep physicians and hospitals from expanding their use of the technology. Also, the lengthy and costly processes to get a license to practice telemedicine, with the ultimate result being restrictive access to service, defeats the existing motivation to move forward with the technology.

Another telemedicine legal issue concerns cross-countries telemedicine licensing. Healthcare providers licensed to practice medicine in one country are limited to treating patients only in their country of residence. Although healthcare providers are generally licensed to practice within certain jurisdictions, telemedicine requires multiple countries licensure, both for their primary country and for the jurisdiction in which services are rendered in order that consistency in treatment is maintained. Further, cross-country licensure will allow patients to continue receiving care from the physician or health provider of their choice and with whom they have established relationship and comfort.

There are different practice requirements across the countries, and the uncertainties related to licensure could be subject to malpractice litigations and ambiguities about how that liability might be addressed; these discrepancies will continue to hinder access to telemedicine.

Therefore, the improvement of existing regulatory laws, along with the proposed creation of cross countries wide telemedicine licenses could ease barriers to medical licensure and telemedicine use in those countries.

- ❖ *Credentialing*

In our observations it was found that the telemedicine credentialing process is complex and requires lengthy transactions. The application procedure for credentialing is a burdensome administrative process requiring time-consuming volumes of forms needing to be submitted. Hence, improving the credentialing procedures via collaborative efforts between each country's governing bodies and the healthcare industry would allow telemedicine providers to request and receive credentialed certifications at any location, removing unnecessary barriers to credentialing and thereby increasing the numbers of providers able to take advantage of telemedicine services.

❖ Health Human Resources

According to our field observation, it was observed that within healthcare provider agencies there were insufficient numbers of professionals and other healthcare workers trained in telemedicine service areas. This shortage in telemedicine savvy providers is another component of the overall shortages in other critical services such as education and general healthcare. The implementation and continued use of Telemedicine can help minimize these shortages as education services can be offered via virtual platforms similar to those used for telemedicine. The overall result would be a trained, educated health workforce capable of navigating the use of telemedicine and delivering quality healthcare service.

❖ *Population Demographics*

There is a general yearly increase in the populations of African countries, the USVI, and Haiti, especially among the young and the elderly. As this increase continues, these nations will face larger numbers within these demographics requiring educational and health care services, especially within the next 30 years. This will place additional stress and burden on existing broken health care systems. Therefore, an urgent focus on telemedicine implementation is needed as it could ease this burden.

❖ *Facility and Service Infrastructure*

This is a significant challenge that severely hampers the ability of African countries, the USVI, and Haiti to improve the health, wellbeing of their populations, and also to decrease expenditures, and enhance patient experiences and quality of care. As of today, many of the physical healthcare structures are in poor condition and existing financial resources and service delivery appears ineffective in both meeting needs and generating revenue.

The physical capacity of laboratories, offices, and equipment are comprised of insufficient staff, reduced financial resources and lack of technical expertise for repair and maintenance, and short supply of medical materials. Many of the current physical healthcare structures were constructed years ago, and improvement delays and increasing maintenance costs are now inhibiting their improvement which affects overall performance and service delivery.

Vulnerabilities in public health service infrastructure have become clearly evident when threats such as HIV/AIDS, Ebola, and the Covid-19 outbreaks resulted in thousands and millions being infected, hospitals not having enough supplies or capacity, laboratories, were flooded with testing samples, and contact tracing efforts were minimal or had major gaps thereby allowing disease even further reach into communities. Many of these general vulnerabilities were well known to governments prior to the diseases rampant march but remain unaddressed due to continuous limited funding resources to remediate them. There is, therefore, an urgent need to address infrastructure improvement along with acquiring necessary technology that can sustain telemedicine services. These improvements must be the primary focus of governments and those responsible for spearheading and allocating finances for healthcare.

A resilient and efficient public health infrastructure is vital not only to act in response to disease outbreaks such as HIV/AIDS, Ebola, and Covid-19, but also to address continuing challenges such as preventing or managing chronic illnesses and controlling recurrent infectious diseases.

- ❖ *Technology and Communications Availability*

Our field observation shows that a larger number of the people in African countries, the USVI, and Haiti are internet users and these countries have equipped access to both priced wireless communication and mobile technology. However, the existing communication infrastructure has limited carrying capacity to channel telemedicine services, which is an important segment for face-to-face consultations between health care providers and patients. Even those who have connectivity and who have a quality-rich mobile device, must work with weak internet network / broadband capacity.

Reduced availability of strong, reliable connectivity, along with computer viruses and restricted capacity remain a constant challenge when and where the Internet is accessible. For telemedicine service functionalities to be effective, internet bandwidth speeds must be in a satisfactory carrying capacity, which includes sufficient audio quality and visual clarity to offer quality health services to the population.

These factors should serve as additional impetus for those in power to introduce and push forward measures and programs to improve technology and communication availability for both the implementation and maintenance of telemedicine and for its expansion throughout the countries so service in congested and rural areas is efficient, resulting in improved patient outcomes.

The conclusion of our interactions with many healthcare providers was that technology and communication availability should be bonded with the medical industry's essential values and with its related benefits.

- ❖ *Health system challenges*

Implementing telemedicine services means merging with existing educational and health care systems if any exist, which requires a comprehensive change of functional capacities. As already stated, telemedicine must be tied to improvements in broadband coverage and connectivity, to government supported and viably funded improvements in physical infrastructure – hospitals, clinics, roads, and equipment, along with vested and targeted actions and policies to bring about improvements in health care performance management and quality.

Health systems should also be coordinated with medical and health education so that providers receive necessary updated training, and information, and credentialing remains current. Universal Health Coverage must be a part of these efforts toward overall improvement and enhancement of existing health systems.

The bottom line is that without concerted and collaborative effort in the aforementioned areas and those discussed throughout this book, health outcomes will continue to be poor and the effectiveness of telemedicine as a partner in bringing about better health relationships and outcomes for both patients and providers will not be realized for these nations.

The first use of telemedicine in the world is said to have been by way of telegraph in 1874 when it was used to manage the care of wounded persons in Australia after an attack on the Barrow Creek Telegraph.[218] Since then, several reports have shown a substantial increase in experience and expertise in the utilization of telemedicine – especially over the last decade in places such as Europe, Canada, the United States, and Japan. Developing countries, including Africa, are equally not strangers to telemedicine. The most interesting evidence on the effectiveness of telemedicine use is presented by the following cases of successful telemedicine projects in Sub-Saharan Africa.

HEALTH NET PROJECTS.

HEALTHNET is one of the most established telemedicine project initiatives in Africa. With the intention of improving the use and practice of telemedicine among health professionals, it has been implemented in 20 countries on the African continent. The system is described as "a computer-based telecommunications system offered by SATELLIFE". It allows for connectivity between and by healthcare specialists worldwide. According to Mbarika and Okoli's, Telemedicine in Sub-Sharan Africa: A Proposed Delphi Study (2003), "SATELLIFE is a charitable organization based in Boston, USA. Using a low earth orbit satellite and phone lines, it provides email access in Sub-Saharan countries, serving over 10,000 healthcare workers. Where adequate telecommunication links exist, SATELLIFE and other organizations offer higher capacity email and internet connections, which allows for sending email attachments such as image files, permitting a form of low-cost telemedicine." [219]

SHARE PROJECT (EAST AFRICA): UGANDA AND KENYA [220]

The primary purpose of Project SHARE was to create audio conference links between clinicians in St. John's, Canada and the Kenyan cities of Kampala and Nairobi with the additional goal of enhancing patient care and medical education at Kampala's Makerere Medical School. The use of satellite networks helped establish the interactive video conference links between the medical facilities in Canada and Kenya.

The SHARE Project is the result of the efforts of two communications organizations, the International Satellite Organization and the International Institute of Communication, which came together in the 1980's with a shared focus to help improve health access in Africa and other developing nations. Together, they created Satellite in Health and Rural Education, which has become known as the SHARE Project.

By establishing satellite links with Nairobi in December 1985 and with Kampala in February 1986, the members of the SHARE Project were able to complete the long-term goal of teaching "Ugandans and Kenyans how to maintain multi-point audio- conferencing technology and design distance education programs." The newly incorporated system was used over a period of "several months for pediatric teaching sessions, administrative meetings, the transmission of electroencephalography (EEGs), and a variety of other applications." According to information provided in Mbarika and Okoli's study, it was pediatricians in St. John's who provided most of the educational programs, "with an additional program hosted by health centers in Ontario and Quebec."

SENEGAL PROJECT [221]

Born out of the collaboration between the Regional University Hospital and the European Institute of Telemedicine in Toulouse, France that encouraged a partnership with health institutions in Senegal, the project aimed to use video-conferencing to conduct telehealth/telemedicine consultations.

The primary components of the project included using video-conferencing, customized for medical use, to conduct in-service distance training for health professionals working in remote health centers. One of the benefits of the project were that three hospitals in the cities of Dakar Fann, St Louis, and

Djourbel were connected by telemedicine links. Using the 'store and forward' method for transmission of data, this linkage permitted the transmission of medical images and other medical information. An advantage of the 'store and forward' data transmission method is that patient data can be transmitted at reduced cost and implemented in phases based upon available financial resources. At the time of the projects' initial roll out the then existing telecommunication network allowed the three hospitals to connect using ISDN lines.

The success of the above project underscores the need for effective approaches to the design and implementation of telemedicine especially as in the case of health and medical services it will be used by and affect a wide broad number and variety of providers and other end-users across continents and countries.

But without continued adequate research and funding, these countries will not meet the utility and economic viability of telemedicine services. No matter how excellently telemedicine services may be presented, unless the ideas and motivation are embraced by all parties, stakeholders, and health care providers, it will not produce the expected results or reach its objectives.

❖ *Training*

Experts acknowledge that implementing telemedicine technology depends on more than just the technical aspects associated with proper broadband ability and electronic medical equipment inter-operability. Telemedicine services also depend on the human element. The most important of these are trained, certified, and qualified community health workers.

The insight of community health workers is of inestimable value for telemedicine success, especially in the delivery of quality medical care to the necessary populations. Qualified and well-trained medical workers are important players for broadening access and providing quality telemedicine services to populations. Yet, in many African countries, the USVI, and Haiti, health care workers lack proper knowledge regarding telemedicine platforms and their usage.

As of now, practical training in virtual care has not been broadly incorporated into medical care services, nursing, or continuing education curricula. Inadequate knowledge and information when working in a new medium or format, causes confusion and uncertainty. Healthcare providers already work under enormous pressure to provide quality care, be knowledgeable, and be considerate of patient needs and expectations while learning and navigating new systems of operation. Therefore, accurate preparation and training of providers, medical schools and teaching hospitals is crucial to successful telemedicine implementation. To help achieve a truly efficacious telemedicine and telehealth system it is imperative that qualified medical education institutions, hospitals and clinics provide mandatory telemedicine courses to staff, future physicians, nurse practitioners, nurses, and other health professionals. Community-based training through education and internet-based/virtual programs would improve the knowledge and abilities of providers to make better use of telemedicine technology to the benefit of health outcomes, overall service delivery, and may prove beneficial for the return on investment.

As innovation in care delivery and technology continue to transform healthcare systems, these countries' authorities must ensure that their current and future healthcare professionals have the tools and resources they need to deliver the best possible care to patients.

❖ *Ensuring sustainability*

Issues surrounding ensuring sustainability of telemedicine services derives from whether African countries, the USVI, and Haitian health providers, in both public and private sectors, will support telemedicine services. Once implemented, support will also be affected by reimbursement through insurance companies, and this remains an uphill issue – especially on the African continent. Another component of sustainability is the maintenance of the systems once in place. There must be technicians trained in the proper upkeep and repair of the system components. The government and/or private companies which own or provide internet services must ensure continued operability and sufficient broadband capacity for telemedicine services to be conducted without interruption.

One way to ensure sustainability from the outset of implementation is by discussing implementation processes with and adapting best practices from practitioners and countries already using telemedicine. This approach could help decide the difference between a sustainable program and a failed one.

Although there are challenges to successful telemedicine implementation, the benefits the technology holds for the healthcare industry are well worth the time and effort. Telemedicine is the future of the healthcare industry and the sooner the healthcare industries of African countries, the USVI, and Haiti address the challenges, the sooner they may reap the benefits of this technology.

- ❖ *Reimbursement challenges through public and private insurance entities*

Despite the prospective benefits telemedicine services can bring, reimbursement through public and private insurance entities and regulatory uncertainty are causing healthcare providers and practitioners to remain doubtful about adopting the technology. Current public and private health insurance mandates and rulings, and patient satisfaction, along with population health management, are also cited as fundamental concerns if the existing regulatory laws remain unchanged.

Like other previously cited challenges, reimbursement policies for telemedicine services through public and private health insurance standards must be improved and amended for healthcare providers to receive remuneration and for the cost of service to be reimbursable and/or affordable for patient users.

Cost to patients and reimbursement or remuneration of providers is a primary factor of concern in developing nations in Africa and the country of Haiti. However, this is also an issue for the USVI where, as a US territory, the average income is just over $37,000 per annum which is $20,000 less than mainland USA states, and 22% of the population lives in poverty.[222, 223]

Hence, the best coverage for telemedicine services may be through the adoption of universal health care that includes proviso for payment to providers. It falls to the responsibility of the governments of these nations to structure regulatory statutes that will provide oversight of insurance companies and provide an outline for payment protocol and to follow this up with measures and mechanisms for enforcement and accountability.

❖ *Surmounting these challenges*

To reduce barriers, studies to ascertain the best telemedicine structure for each country and its urban and rural areas should be conducted. Discussions as to what sources will finance the cost of implementation and maintenance, broadband enhancements, actual equipment, and software for telemedicine platforms should be at the forefront of government and agency planning. Simultaneously, regulations to oversee confidentiality, privacy, access, and accountability must be established.

There are some compelling examples of this type of pre-planning and strategizing taking place throughout the world. However, for such efforts to be effective and for telemedicine to become mainstream, all stakeholders and government must be motivated to embrace telemedicine either because of its substantial potential to be a core part of the health care delivery system infrastructure, or due to its ability to leverage a strong lever to bend the cost curve and make these countries healthcare system easier to navigate.

Telemedicine is the future of healthcare systems, and the sooner government representatives and health care providers address the challenges, the sooner they may reap its benefits.

CHAPTER FOUR:
ADDITIONAL APPLICATIONS OF TELEMEDICINE

PART 1:
HEALTHCARE PROVIDER SHORTAGE

Healthcare provider shortages and related problems are making it harder for individuals, especially those residing in a distant community to visit a physician. There is also the persistent shortfall affecting people, facilities, and industries outside healthcare's normal reach. As direct repercussions, the disrupted healthcare systems incur longer waitlists, have more burned-out providers, experience reduced patient involvement, and see greater risks to the health of patients.

Existing trends reveal that these conditions will continue and even worsen, causing substantial negative effects on the quality of health and healthcare services delivery.

World Health Organization published reports estimate that 57 countries, including the USVI and Haiti, have a clear shortage of more than 2.3 million doctors, nurses, and midwives, resulting in an inequitable ratio of healthcare workers to citizens which further increases the lack of adequate capacity to provide significant health interventions.[224] Other reports state that these two nations and African countries are estimated to have fewer than one doctor per 1000 people compared to 10 per 1000 in developed countries. [225]

Physician shortage is defined by the World Health Organization (WHO) as having fewer than 80 percent of the physicians required to meet provider demand and, as a minimal provision, as having one doctor for every 1,000 residents of a geographical area. [226, 227]

Unfortunately, these areas do not meet these criteria. Instead, they are still showing an average ratio of ten doctors per 100,000 residents which makes it difficult to provide access to quality healthcare services. It is further reported that the shortage is primarily due to the incapacity of governments to invest in the training of healthcare providers, which over years produces not only scarcity in the number of specialists but also primary care physicians and contributes to a disappointing healthcare service delivery system.[228]

Although few countries have attempted to focus on the urgent shortfall of healthcare providers, the intricacy and scope of this problem make it challenging to solve. The perseverance of the shortage as it is presented today, is also due to a continuing brain drain – the lure of medical, scientific, and IT graduates and specialists to more developed nations. This brain drain is costing a loss in the billions of dollars for African nations. [229, 230]

Another issue in the healthcare provider shortage is the of lack of effective financial resources to meet even modest salary demands. The pervasive paucity of adequate remuneration for their services, results in many qualified healthcare providers leaving medicine altogether and seeking other professions, leaving public health services, and going into more lucrative private practice, or emigrating to other countries or continents where remuneration, work conditions, incentives and other opportunities may be superior. Other physicians and health workers in these countries are underemployed or unemployed. [231, 232]

The previously mentioned brain drain of Africa's medical and scientific talent is benefitting many neighboring countries and continents such as South

Africa, the Dominican Republic, Europe, the Caribbean, and North America. The loss of highly skilled professionals has deleterious effects on African countries, the USVI, Haiti and other developing nations.[233-237]

The shortage of healthcare providers is further aggravated by evidence that authorities in the areas have become overly dependent on unqualified national and foreign health workers. This dependency has fashioned a process wherein instead of improving current healthcare organizations to educate, train, and supply a larger qualified professional labor workforce, they instead, promote a practice of anticipation and demand for unqualified national and foreign assistance to provide relief to ailing and faulty functioning health systems.[238] A pragmatic remedy to this problem would be to increase healthcare specialty training and create an organizational environment that will contribute to retaining successful healthcare specialists. Such actions are an imperative that requires long-term solution – strategizing and commitment from governments.

In suggesting this approach, it is important that governments and healthcare providers understand staffing shortages within the medical field, are both a quantitative and a qualitative problem that must be addressed in order to have a queue of skilled, knowledgeable, and qualified medical and other health workers.

The modern medical environment associated with current health inequality requires providers to focus, not only on primary agents that lead to sicknesses, but also to discuss societal determinant factors of health such as poverty, inequity, unawareness, and population exclusion and disenfranchisement.[239, 240]

If public health systems are to be enhanced and improved, it is crucial to find innovative strategies beneficial to the population and the health workforce, along with strengthening mechanisms and practices for ensuring better productivity and accountability.

PART 2:
HEALTH SUB-SPECIALTIES THAT ADD VALUE IN HEALTHCARE PROVIDER SHORTAGE

As the projected shortage of physicians and specialists continues to be a growing concern, the governments of African countries, the USVI, and Haiti should take full advantage of the development of virtual healthcare services outside the range of normal primary care service delivery. The advent, improvements, and expansion of telemedicine platforms have opened the possibility for an unprecedented upsurge of new telemedicine specialties in using the components of video consultations, data sharing, or remote monitoring. While these specialty platforms may not be an effective solution for some surgical fields, they may, however, prove to be a practical opportunity and means of easing the persistent shortage of primary care and physician specialists for other medical areas and specialties.

To narrow the gaps created by socioeconomic and health disparities and inequities demands exploration of diverse approaches to providing access to quality healthcare services along with implementing effective tools that can benefit and meet desired outcomes of neglected populations. Telemedicine and its many medical platforms and specialties offer a wide range of innovative approaches which, when implemented and incorporated into existing healthcare systems, can expand provider-patient engagement, ease the burden of physician-patient travel, allow for continued and accessible health and welfare monitoring, follow-up, diagnosis, and evaluation, and can be an available solution to the physician and specialist shortage.

The sections below present a few telemedicine specialties which can be incorporated into healthcare systems to provide neglected communities access to quality health services across a broad range of medical practices.

TELERADIOLOGY [241-243]

Access to radiologists presents a significant problem for patients residing in remote areas as specialists and equipment to perform radiography and radiographic procedures are not readily available. Compounding lack of availability is that technicians qualified to perform repair and maintenance of radiological equipment tend not to be as available in rural areas. The insufficiency of radiology specialists further adds to the problems of accessibility and radiological service delivery.

In light of those considerations, teleradiology has become an essential platform for delivering rural and remote populations the exceptional level of care they deserve. Teleradiology will improve access to care by allowing radiologists the ability to offer their expertise without being present with the individual, and also without the patient having to travel to receive services. This could be a significant factor since most radiological specialists (MRI, pediatric, and neuro-radiologists) are always needed in inaccessible locations and are available only during daytime hours in urban areas.

Teleradiology services are designed to increase access to radiographic images such as X-rays or CT scans from distant locations with the support of an on-site care provider. Overall, teleradiology appears to be a practical and sustainable answer to the recurrent shortage of subspecialty radiology care in rural and remote locations.

TELEPSYCHIATRY [244-246]

A shortage of competent psychiatrists has been a continuous problem for the last two decades. Using psychiatric telemedicine can be viewed as an effective alternative solution to both the initial consultation and follow-up patient encounter compared to conventional in-person approaches and can ease the decline of quality access to behavioral health benefits.

The lack of experienced psychiatrists has compelled primary healthcare providers to prescribe therapeutic medicines as the first line of treatment, which places them in a problematic light if there are medication blunders. As new psychotropic medicines are recommended and prescribed to mental health patients, primary care physicians are less inclined to continue prescribing these medications and are not sufficiently knowledgeable in mental and behavioral health issues and therapies to continue the mandatory psychotherapy and follow-up services. Hence, psychiatric telemedicine can empower competent psychiatrists to offer diagnosis and therapy to more patients, including people with restricted flexibility such as the aged, prisoners, and those lacking transportation or physically unable to travel to urban areas.

Another bonus of telepsychiatry services is, they have increased patient interaction. This may be because patients are within the comfort of their homes and thus avoid the stigma some cultures associate with seeking psychiatric help. Thus, overall, telepsychiatry has the propensity to enhance access to psychological and psychiatric services in a more affordable and accessible manner.

TELECARDIOLOGY [247-249] AND TELE-PULMONOLOGY [250-255]

In this book, these two telemedicine specialties are presented together because cardiac and pulmonary diseases and conditions can affect both systems in the human body.

Cardiologists, cardiac specialties, and pulmonologists are experiencing a severe shortage with harmful impacts on the health of the populations of the USVI, Haiti, and nations in Africa. Implementing and extending tele- cardiology/pulmonary services, especially to rural and remote areas, will not only provide the opportunity to lessen the negative shortage but will also improve the way cardiac and pulmonary care are delivered in urban and distant primary care locations.

Every year, millions in Africa, the USVI, and Haiti die from cardiovascular and pulmonary diseases such as arterial hypertension, stroke, cardiomyopathies, rheumatic heart disease, chronic obstructive pulmonary disease (COPD), asthma, bronchitis, and other upper respiratory illnesses primarily due to a lack of focus on cardiovascular and pulmonary diseases. [279, 280] Peer-reviewed and other professional reports show that cardiovascular diseases account for over 10% of adult hospital admissions yearly, and 7% from heart failure, while the incidence of asthma and other pulmonary diseases have increased, especially in adults aged 18-55 years.[256-259] Cardiovascular diseases are now classified as a public health problem requiring immediate focus and solutions. [260]

Although actual morbidity related to cardiovascular diseases is less in poorer countries, mortality is markedly higher due to deteriorated healthcare infrastructure, lack of access to quality health services and medications, and the cost of transportation from distanced rural localities to hospitals or doctor's offices.[261-263]

In the USVI, Haiti, and many African nations, the morbidity and mortality rates due to cardiovascular and pulmonary diseases are rising, yet this significant impact is not regarded as a health priority by several governments of these countries.[264-265]

Excessive mortality is aggravated by the total absence of responsiveness of governments and policymakers, and the persistent shortage of pulmonology and cardiovascular specialists capable of performing spirometry, pulmonary function tests, interventional cardiology, cardiac catheterization, cardiac surgery, and to authorize and initiate proper post-surgical follow-up treatments.

Therefore, to address this persistent critical issue, a concerted approach to the overall improvement of healthcare systems and infrastructure, along with targeted programs and incentives to reduce physician and medical specialty shortages must be developed via a collaborative effort between providers, government, other stakeholders, and financial backers. Tele-cardiology/pulmonology are a major and necessary part of these approaches as they will provide an opportunity to grow the scope of these much-needed services and help to create an integrated extension of a network of specialists, thereby strengthening and restructuring current delivery.

TELEDERMATOLOGY [266-267]

Teledermatology platforms can prospectively bridge the gap between affordability and accessibility by offering a rapid path for remote consultation to improve and treat skin diseases and conditions.

Teledermatology can empower primary healthcare providers and patients to interconnect with a dermatologist for diagnosis and treatment of a rash, a mole, or other skin anomalies via visual (including photographs and viewing via phone or computer screen) and data communication or audio. This will allow the dermatologist to render a diagnosis and treatment plan, and the patient can receive guidance on the best remedy to be used and the treatment regimen to be followed. Furthermore, it can be used as a source of educational material for training, and dermatologic curriculum for healthcare providers, and public health education of communities.

During COVID-19, recommendations to use Teledermatology were made by the American Medical Association and the American Dermatological Association as a means of minimizing risk for the elderly and those residing in rural communities.

TELEOPHTHALMOLOGY [268-270]

Teleophthalmology platforms appear to be an effective alternative path to provide needed and prompt care for retinopathy of prematurity (ROP), ophthalmic disease screening, diagnosis and monitoring, and suitable recommendations and/or referrals to other experts. Studies have found that teleophthalmology visits are just as effective for diagnoses, management, and monitoring of patients who have ROP, DR, and age-related macular degeneration (ARMD), and patient satisfaction was rated as high as ninety-eight percent.

Although it may be in the early stages of development in these countries, the full implementation and use of Teleophthalmology platforms will also empower ophthalmologists to offer screening and referral for diabetic retinopathy (DR), glaucoma, age-related macular degeneration (ARMD), and other vision diseases. One of the operative benefits of teleophthalmology is that it enables images of the quality fundus to be stored in a protected server and transferred to selected ophthalmologists, who can then provide an adequate diagnostic for follow-up treatment.

These platforms use the store-and-forward process, supported by interactive functions and remote monitoring processes. They are known to give similar high clinical satisfaction levels and appropriateness as in-person consultations.

TELENEPHROLOGY [271-275]

Chronic kidney disease (CKD) continues to be a serious health concern with major impacts upon the quality of life, especially in Africa where between 4.9 million and 9.7 million people require treatment for CKD, and at least two million die due to inaccessibility of treatment. Dialysis centers are few and far between and are expensive. Further complicating the possibility of treatment options is that facilities and specialists qualified to perform kidney transplantation are severely limited in supply. The development of practical strategies to ease patients suffering from chronic kidney disease is undermined by a shortage of nephrology specialists combined with geographical distance, which adds trauma and additional expense.

A pressing necessity for innovative approaches that can deliver health services capable of meeting quality standards is imperative if decreasing the number of fatalities caused by recurring kidney infection and CKD is a desired health outcome (as it should be). Using Telenephrology platforms may help to decrease the shortage of nephrologists and enhance the quality of access to healthcare delivery systems to persons residing in remote and/or marginalized communities.

Telenephrology, a key component of telehealth in kidney care, is proven to deliver effective diagnosis and treatment of various glomerular pathologies with results similar to those provided by in office visits. Failure to incorporate and use Telenephrology platforms in healthcare systems will only further contribute to inequities in access, quality, and costs of kidney care services for the most marginalized populations.

TELEOBSTETRICS [276-280]

Despite a collaborative effort to improve reproductive health services and decrease the impact of various maternal risk factors among women, there is still an urgent necessity to offer creativity, and provide better access and quality health management to pregnant women.

According to a peer review conducted by the WHO covering the period 2000 to 2017 and released in 2019, it was found that 94% of all maternal deaths occur in low and middle-income countries. Adolescents and teenagers between the ages of 10-19 are known to experience greater risks of complications and death due to pregnancy. Of the 295,000 deaths resulting from pregnancy in 2017, 196,000 occurred in African nations. Unfortunately, this higher rate of maternal deaths among teenagers echoes the persistent healthcare disparities and heightened financial burden affecting those living in rural and remote areas; factors which are substantiated by the report.

In order to address and decrease maternal deaths and disparities in healthcare entails not only improving the quality of health care access but also incorporating substantial initiatives designed to complement existing healthcare delivery systems that are focused on improving health outcomes pre, during, and post-pregnancy. Teleobstetrics offers a comprehensive pathway for improving access, quality, and cost-effectiveness by adding services and resolving the shortage of prenatal care specialists by increasing their availability via the telemedicine/Teleobstetrics platform.

Included in Teleobstetrics are ultrasounds, fetal echocardiography, psychiatry, diabetes, infectious disease, postpartum depression, gestational diabetes, hypertension, and preeclampsia. The technology allows obstetricians to review test outcomes, monitor symptoms, and view and develop medication and treatment plans, deliver post-operative care, and offer family planning services from distant locations. Female adolescents, teenagers, and adult women could receive obstetric services through their primary doctor, health center offices, and homes without on-site appointments.

TELEONCOLOGY/HEMATOLOGY

Teleoncology platforms, which include pathology, and radiology, are used to amplify screening, diagnosis, therapies, and palliative care.

According to the GLOBOCAN 2018 database, African countries are experiencing an increase in cancer deaths (7.3%,) because of critical factors such as disparities in healthcare services, and limited access to early detection and treatment.[281] Additionally, medical and scientific peer-reviewed studies have found that infection-related cancers in African countries account for 33 percent of all cases and half a million Africans die of cancer each year due to inaccessibility to effective treatment. [282-283]

Much of this increase is not only because deterrence and early diagnostic strategies and approaches are either non-existent or inappropriate, but also financial resources for healthcare services and expertise to mitigate the negative impacts are insufficient or unavailable.[284] Evidence from the WHO suggests the shortfall of healthcare specialists and infrastructure, along with impractical cancer monitoring strategies, are disturbing and have unfairly prevented rural and remote localities from enjoying effective healthcare services.[285]

Teleoncology platforms have shown the possibility of improving both access and quality of cancer care treatment through the use of store-and-forward telemedicine technologies. [286]

Incorporating Teleoncology services into the healthcare industry may help reduce cancer care disparities among the poor and provide an opportunity to ensure accessibility and standards of quality for inexpensive cancer medications are met.

TELEPATHOLOGY

Telepathology services offer a supplemental pathway to supply remote primary diagnostic, second assessment appointment, quality support, research, and education through store-and-forward high-resolution images and videos in support-restricted areas. Only on the medical scene since 1986, telepathology surgeons and pathologist are successfully using it. Comparative literature studies substantiate that when used by surgeons taking tissue samples (such as a biopsy), telepathology reduces the time delay between retrieving the sample and diagnosis. From a financial perspective, this service is of considerable benefit to hospitals and clinics in both urban and rural areas. The service has been shown to reduce the cost of a dedicated pathologist because telepathology services are available via the internet and telehealth modules, thus negating the need for travel and the need to have pathologists on-site at each clinic/hospital. [287]

The implementation and support of telepathology platforms are an innovative approach to supplement the shortage of competent pathology specialists and improve access to quality health for neglected populations. Telepathology can make possible collaborative relationships and significant scientific opportunities for hospitals and academic institutions. Each of the primary telepathology platforms –static image-based systems, virtual slide systems, real-time systems, and whole slide imaging (WSI) can be managed remotely, thereby enhancing access and reducing cost. [288]

TELEREHABILITATION

According to the United Nations Department of Economic and Social Affairs yearly report (2010), the African continent accounts for 63% of the population in rural and remote areas, and those lacking access to effective and quality healthcare specialties compared to those living in major urban metropolises.[289]

Although current data on the exact number of healthcare therapists are inadequate, the World Health Organization (2006) reports that these areas are facing a substantial shortfall of four (4) million healthcare specialists. This dearth of medical professionals is expected to increase as the African population is predicted to grow by 2050. [290, 291]

Incorporation of Telerehabilitation platforms, which include therapeutic interventions, monitoring of improvement, education, consultation, training, and networking, appears to be a conceivable avenue of supplementing the critical shortfall of competent specialists in physiotherapy specialties, especially in rural and remote localities. Telerehabilitation will not only allow competent therapists to engage with patients remotely and provide access to quality rehabilitation services, but it can also serve as an effective network through which mentoring and support can be given to healthcare providers in rural and remote areas.

The expansion of Telerehabilitation will provide people living in underserved areas a sense of autonomy, which will empower them to invest in their healthcare management and decrease the negative impact of socioeconomic factors related to healthcare expenditures.

TELE-ENDOCRINOLOGY

Implementation and expansion of tele-endocrinology services will lessen unnecessary travel expenses of physicians and patients. It will help ensure the population has access to specialty endocrinology providers who can diagnose and treat conditions such as diabetes, thyroid disease, and osteoporosis or metabolic bone illness. Studies verify that patients receiving services via tele-endocrinology have at least a 17% improvement in Hemoglobin A1c; 70% of patients had improvements in dyslipidemia, and 97% said they were pleased with the virtual care services provided.[292]

Tele-endocrinology services will fill the vacuum when a lack of endocrinology specialists disrupts normal provider-patient experiences and will provide continued consultations, monitor patients, and refill prescriptions.

TELENEUROLOGY

A continuing shortfall in the availability of qualified neurologists for the diagnosis and treatment of neurologic disorders continues to be a persistent cause of disability and death, especially in rural and remote localities.[293]

The Global Burden of Disease annual report states that although stroke is classified as a leading cause of mortality and morbidity, migraine, meningitis, dementia, and epilepsy are also huge causes of disability, particularly in underprivileged populations where effective efforts to provide quality access to neurosurgical services have proven challenging.

Other published reports state that in 1998 the African continent had 500 neurosurgeons; an average of one for every 1,350,000 inhabitants within a distance of 70,000 km^2; by 2001 the number of neurosurgeons had increased by 65.[294-296] The WHO reports that the number of specialists in neurology in Africa, at 0.03 per 100,000 population, is lower than in other WHO regions.[297]

Haiti, however, presents a different picture. The country of 10.5 million people has far fewer specialists to address the enormous burden of neurological conditions. Currently, there are only four (4) neurosurgeons practicing in Haiti, and all practice within the city of Port-au-Prince, limiting the amount of care they can provide to Haitians outside of the capital. The neurosurgeon ratio per 100,000 people is only about 0.04, and there is no structured model of neurosurgical care beyond the city limits of Port-au-Prince.[298, 299]

As of right now, we do not have data available to understand fully how the shortage of neurosurgeons in the USA is impacting or will impact the population in the United States Virgin Islands. It is important to note that we faced significant limitations with collecting workforce shortage data for the U.S. Virgin Islands because healthcare systems are yet recovering from hurricane damage.

The United States mainland is said to have an increasing shortage of neurosurgeons dating back to 2012. Unlike other medical specialty areas whose shortages are due to brain drain and just low numbers, the dearth of neurosurgeons is tied directly to the arduous education necessary to acquire proficiency in this specialty. Including undergraduate and graduate medical education, it generally takes 7 years to produce a fully trained neurosurgeon. In the USA neurosurgery residency trains 1200 candidates annually and graduates half that number. Coupled with the rigors of the program is the fact that fewer medical school graduates choose neurosurgery due to its long training, onerous malpractice insurance, high caseload (because they are in short supply), and long work hours.[300, 301]

There are over 5,700 hospitals in the United States with less than 3,700 neurosurgeons, and more recent analyses place the current ratio at around 1:61,000. With a growing and aging population, it seems this proportion may still be inadequate in meeting current health care needs.[302]

As the USVI is a territory of the United States, and many of its physicians train on the mainland, it is not presumptive to assert that the shortage in the neurosurgery workforce the mainland United States is facing is being felt more strongly in the U.S. Virgin Islands.

These factors show a critical lack of available neurologists in these countries, which affects the population's ability to access quality neurological services.

The rapid development of Teleneurology in more developed nations is providing countless opportunities to enhance neurological services to neglected populations. Therefore, based on these findings, incorporating Teleneurology platforms will give neurologists the capacity and ability to offer services at a distance to those residing in inaccessible locations. Teleneurology can also help decrease the effects of provider shortage, as it will enable a single neurologist to treat more patients in various locations with minimal increases in overhead and staffing costs, thus making its incorporation a cost-effective measure. The enhanced availability would mean diagnosis, treatment, and follow-up care for stroke, seizure disorders, and other neurological maladies could be conducted efficiently without additional burden to patient or provider.

TELEGASTROENTEROLOGY

Gastroenterological illnesses (diarrheal disease, hepatitis B, and H. pylori), rates of morbidity and mortality continue to be outstanding medical issues in disenfranchised populations and underserved communities, especially among infants and children.

Despite growths in economic developments of some African countries and Haiti, unclean water, futile urbanization, housing, and improper hygiene and sanitation systems are the foremost contributing factors to persistent increases in gastroenterological infections. Only 34% of inhabitants of less developed and poor nations have suitable sanitation, and specifically in sub-Saharan Africa, more than 40% of the population lack access to safe and clean water. [303] The result of all these factors is a surge in the pervasiveness of gastroenterological illnesses such as gallbladder and digestive cancers becoming a serious public health issue.

The need to build a strong supply of specialists in gastroenterology to form a vital clinical and research specialty area is needed. But, as in most specialties, there is a significant shortfall of specialists to provide access to quality gastroenterology health services to the underserved population, especially in rural and remote localities. Africa, alone, needs a projected 1.5 million more healthcare providers just to offer primary health services to its populations. [304] Yet, for the last past decades, several governments of African countries and Haiti have not been including and sustaining training of gastroenterology specialists in their financial commitment.[305]

As with the preceding telehealth specialties, incorporating Telegastroenterology into the existing healthcare system is the most efficacious means of achieving a broad scope and availability of care for all citizens.

With Telegastroenterology platforms remote populations can access services without traveling outside their neighborhoods, thus receiving medical expertise through on-site consultations. Another advantage of this virtual approach is that it enables collaboration between the gastroenterologist and the primary care provider, thereby fostering better patient follow-up and diminished cost.

People facing gastroenterological illnesses such as diarrheal disease, hepatitis B, and H pylori and chronic conditions as Crohn's disease, hepatitis C, and colitis need monitoring and assistance, making Telegastroenterology platforms an excellent choice for gastroenterology practices.

TELEUROLOGY

Consistent with the other medical specialty areas, the burden of urological diseases and conditions, such as urologic cancers (prostate cancer is one type), urinary incontinence, acute and chronic urinary tract infections, urethral injuries, fertility evaluation, and problems interrelated to reproductive organs is persistent and pervasive. These diseases and conditions can have critical impacts on population health; and unfortunately, consistent with most of the telemedicine medical specialties already mentioned, there is a shortage of urologists in developed and developing nations, thereby limiting access to proper care. Similar to neurosurgery, a major contributing factor to the shortage of urologists is training. It has been suggested that telemedicine may be used to supplement traditional training methods – especially in the COVID-19 pandemic.[306] In addition to lengthy and difficult training, the average age of urologists is said to be 53; thus, more are departing the field faster than new ones are entering. The impact of this loss is greatest and hardest upon rural areas where often disease is rampant and the need, extensive.[307]

Added to the issues of shortage and loss is that the remaining urological workforce suffers serious burnout due to patient overload and indeterminate long work hours. The persistent shortage of urology specialists is a substantial problem that seriously diminishes the available supply of doctors compelled to encounter and provide suitable solutions to the rising health service needs of African countries, the USVI, and Haiti.[308] Therefore, addressing these challenges requires governments and healthcare providers of these countries to understand the urological significance and adopt new clinical approaches, primary among which is telemedicine.

As the populations of African, USVI, and Haiti continue to grow and age, the availability of urologists will be even more of a critical factor. The use of telemedicine can help relieve the burden of urological impacts. Already being used in the United States, it has been found that patient satisfaction is high, and expected health outcomes have not diminished or been negatively affected. The satisfaction of patients is a significant component in measuring the effectiveness of service; TeleUrology can enhance that satisfaction and increase access to quality care.

Tele-urology platforms offer realistic benefits such as diagnosis, treatment of acute and chronic urinary tract, pre-and post-operative care, second opinions, and remote post-operative follow-up treatment. Furthermore, the tele-urology platforms offer the opportunity to decrease the financial burden of out-of-pocket expenditures, the extensive waiting list for scheduled medical procedures, underfunding services, and patient transportation to health facilities.

Access to quality healthcare services for most of the neglected is contingent on improved high-quality urological care, therefore, incorporating and implementing this approach must be a key priority.

TELERHEUMATOLOGY

Despite many initiatives to decrease the hardship impact, the rheumatological disease continues to cause chronic morbidity within the population. According to the Global Burden of Disease report (2010), rheumatic and musculoskeletal diseases have been recognized as the second leading cause of disability as compared by years lived with incapacity.[309-311]

Some of the reasons are insufficient healthcare resources, a persistent shortage of health professional workforce, delayed diagnosis arising from poor education, inadequate financial budgeting, misappropriation of funds, undernourishment, unclean water, hygiene, poverty, and limited access to quality healthcare services. Furthermore, the occurrence of persistent chronic morbidity has been overstretching healthcare provider's capacities which are already struggling with a critical shortage of specialists to cope with the growing frequency of rheumatological diseases (rheumatoid arthritis, juvenile idiopathic arthritis, gout, myositis to systemic lupus erythematosus, and antiphospholipid syndrome).

To cope with these challenges, incorporating TeleRheumatology platforms into existing health systems in developed nations has shown effective results in facilitating access to quality healthcare provider specialties, and enhanced diagnosis and management of rheumatology diseases, especially in remote and rural areas. Of great benefit is that it has been reported that TeleRheumatology health outcomes and diagnosis are both precise, and satisfactory to healthcare providers and patients, and are cost-effective.

Incorporating and implementing TeleRheumatology will decrease the disproportion and paucity of healthcare services, and provide equitable access to specialties such as rheumatologists, orthopedic surgeons, physical medicine and rehabilitation, occupational therapists, and physiotherapists, which contribute to the mitigation of the disease and improves population well-being.

GERIATRIC TELEMEDICINE

As the numbers of an aging population, coupled with the persistent hardship of chronic disease explodes, many developing countries still lack effective human and healthcare infrastructures with devoted resources and services to meit the growing needs.

It is estimated that by 2050 the elderly of Africa over 65 years of age will account for as much as 10% of the overall population, a substantial increase from the 4.5% projected for 2030, and an even more dramatic increase from 3.6% in 2010. [312] In the USVI, those 65 and older constitute just over 19% of the current population; [313] while in Haiti the current 65 and older population is approximately 5% with 589,966 people in that category; this demographic is anticipated to increase by 2030 to 6.1% with 803,643 elderly requiring readily available access to care for chronic conditions. These facts are of major consequence in consideration of the fact that non-communicable diseases account for 57% of all deaths in Haiti.[314,315]

As of today, African countries, USVI, and Haiti are not prioritizing geriatrics in their medical programs, resulting in a critical lack of geriatricians to provide access to quality healthcare services for the elderly population. In consideration of these facts' limited resources, there is a tremendous need to explore alternative approaches designed to offer comprehensive gerontological healthcare services, especially those living in rural and remote localities where many elderly tend to retire in these countries.

One of the best approaches for decreasing this gap would be the incorporation and implementation of the geriatric telemedicine platforms - a safe, convenient way for distant geriatricians to provide access and quality care. Gerontological telemedicine services have been demonstrated to be effective and comparable to face-to-face visits, have great diagnostic reliability, enhance interrelation with a healthcare provider, and patient satisfaction.

Remote geriatricians can use the geriatric telemedicine services to watch and consult the aging population in the comfort of their homes using home-monitoring equipment, resulting in decreasing needless travel and hospital cost.

Overall, the use of the Geriatric Telemedicine services within African countries, USVI, and Haiti healthcare system will provide endless opportunities for healthcare providers to develop a new standard of commitment to the aging population.

TELE-GYNECOLOGY

Although the maternal mortality rate has been showing signs of decline in developing countries, complications during childbearing and pregnancy in African countries, USVI, and Haiti, however, continue to pose an unnecessary risk and claim the lives of women. Worldwide, in 2017, approximately 295,000 women died during and after pregnancy and childbirth; two-thirds of those women (196,000) were in Sub-Saharan Africa. Most maternal deaths are correlated to inequitable access to quality health services and are especially acute for poorer women. Haiti is among the 15 nations the WHO has placed on 'high alert' as a fragile state wherein maternal mortality is a critical health issue; 10 of the countries are in Africa.[316]

It has been recognized that complications through delivery and pregnancy are among the major determinants of death and more than half of motherly losses occur two weeks after post-delivery because of childbirth-related health problems varying from postnatal hemorrhage to sepsis and hypertensive illnesses. Not only are mothers affected, but newborns also: 4 million babies die within the first month of delivery – primarily in underdeveloped countries.[317-319]

Most women and their unborn children have been recognized not only to lack access to basic healthcare services such as detection, prevention, and treatment of severe complications but also to quality obstetric healthcare specialties because of the continuing shortage of obstetricians and gynecologists (OB-GYNs). With 24% of the world's disease burden, Africa also has the most alarming shortage of healthcare workers caused by deprived work environments, aging health workforce, insufficient availability of medical education, and outmigration (brain drain) to other countries.[320] Additional factors such as staffing and retention policies, inadequate funding, international migration, career changes among health workers, premature retirement, morbidity, and premature mortality are also seriously contributing factors to the persistent healthcare provider shortage in African countries, USVI, and Haiti.[321- 323]

In consideration of these facts, the health improvement of women's and children's access to quality OBGYN services necessitates a novel approach to the prenatal, delivery, and post-natal process. A probable positive approach for coping with critical high-burden issues is the incorporation and implementation of the Tele-gynecologist platforms within the health systems. In some countries a tele-gynecology program called the EVA Teleconsultation can connect clinicians in different places – one at the point of care; the other in another location - so that the senior or more skilled clinician can guide the other through examinations, patient consultations, etc. in real-time.[324] This telemedicine technology can provide options for enhancing and increasing the availability of practitioners, training, and other needed services, and can be of exceptional benefit to women and girls residing in remote and poorer communities.

Uses of tele-gynecology technology may include consultations and diagnosis of postpartum depression, gestational diabetes, hypertension, and preeclampsia, family planning services, reviewing test results, monitoring symptoms medication plans, and delivering post-operative care via remote technology.

Some may argue against this approach because of the usual hands-on nature of gynecological and obstetric visits and consultations; however, studies have been conducted, and guidelines to render the most effective services and gain the best health outcomes have been developed. One such study denotes in order to overcome and address disparities in rural and urban gynecological care, four modalities may be employed:

- ❖ Live video, which uses audiovisual telecommunications technology.
- ❖ Store-and-forward, which involves the transmission of health information such as x-rays and other images through a secure electronic communications system to a healthcare provider.
- ❖ Remote patient monitoring, which involves the electronic transmission of health data from a patient in one location to a provider in another location: and

❖ Mobile health (mHealth), which includes healthcare and education supported by mobile devices such as tablets and cell phones

The aforementioned methods are considered both convenient and cost-effective means of providing specialty and subspecialty care that may not be locally available; and telehealth can be used for high-risk and low-risk pregnancies, in gynecology, and for routine and specialty examinations. It has been demonstrated that telehealth results in lower costs overall to healthcare systems, less travel is required by patient and providers, and there is reduced emergency room usage. In use for pregnancy prenatal follow-up, outcomes between traditional in-person visits and telemedicine consultations have been similar. High-risk pregnancy patients have also been shown to benefit immensely from telehealth services, especially when accessible transportation is an issue, or transporting the mother-to-be may increase her risk. When used in rural areas, the on-site rural practitioner can continue overseeing the care of patients while receiving direction from a remotely situated specialist via teleconsultation; and physical examination of high-risk persons can be carried out via videoconferencing between the specialist and the on-site physician.[325]

In consideration of the enormous loss of life among mothers and neonates, the use of tele-gynecology/obstetrics must be at the table of discussion for improvements and enhancements to existing healthcare systems in Africa, the USVI, and Haiti.

TELEAUDIOLOGY

Most of the 32 million children with hearing loss live in low-income and middle-income nations -many of which are in Southeast Asia and Sub-Saharan Africa. [326,329]

However, specific data as to the types and decibel levels of hearing loss have been difficult to gather as many African nations do not track such data, a standardized method for measuring hearing impairment and loss has not been developed and causes of hearing impairment are not tracked.

At least 60% of childhood hearing loss is preventable. For children, hearing loss and impairment can affect speech and language acquisition, academic and social development. Furthermore, hearing impaired and challenged children are more likely to suffer abuse, are at higher risk of injury, endure psychological and emotional consequences of severe loneliness, isolation, anger, and self-esteem issues.[330]

One of the key factors in determining the impact of hearing loss and impairment, aside from age of onset, degree or severity of hearing loss, age at which the loss or impairment is identified, and at which intervention takes place, is the environment. For the children of Sub-Saharan Africa, the environment is critical as it determines access to medical care – urgent and non-urgent, cultural responses and considerations to those with hearing diseases, access to interventions, technology to mitigate and even remediate hearing loss.

Although genetics can have a role in hearing dysfunction, some of the primary culprits are noise and common childhood diseases that go untreated, do not receive proper treatment, or are not treated in sufficient time to prevent long-lasting damage. These illnesses include rubella, cytomegalovirus, mumps, meningitis (responsible for 25% of cases of deafness in some African countries) [331] measles, and chronic ear infections, otitis media, bacterial infections, and lack of hygiene.[332-333]

In addition, the lack of effective awareness education of hearing impairment within the community population and the tenacious shortage of healthcare specialists continues to affect the everyday life of those affected with hearing loss.

Research and studies of current audiological medical practices that employ Teleaudiology platforms have shown that audiologists can provide hearing aid programming remotely, along with conducting remote evaluations and assessments.[334]

Teleaudiology has also been found to be compliant with what is known as the self-fit product market wherein a patient can fit and program their hearing device entirely independently. With Teleaudiology self-fit products can be delivered and set up in an omni-channel or blended service model in which the patient/product client can interface with the audiological clinic and online services for purchase and fitting of devices and get support.[335]

Modern advancements in Teleaudiology techniques and technology have made it possible for audiologists to conduct hearing assessments, fitting of hearing appliances, and can do so with guidance from a senior audiological specialist or clinician.[336] The ear canal and the concha can be scanned, providing a 3-D image, and transmitted to another clinician, diagnostician, or hearing device manufacturer in less than two minutes, eliminating shipping costs and time delays due to mail systems. Cochlear implant tele-consultations have been performed and have post cochlear implant follow-up examinations and have proven to be reliable alternative processes to the traditional in-office visit.[337]

All these advances can be of particular benefit to improving access to and quality of care, diagnosis, and continued treatment of children and adults suffering from ear infections, hearing loss, and impairment. Teleaudiology services will be of special benefit in rural areas where insufficient numbers of audiologists and lack of access to audiological equipment are major limiting factors to care and the remediation of disease. It is not presumptuous to state that if African nations implement tele-audiological services and combine that with increased and enhanced education and educational opportunities, improvements in sanitation and water quality, and establish in-school testing programs, the prevalence and incidence of hearing loss and impairment among the people of Sub-Saharan Africa may decrease.

Haiti has recognized the incidence of hearing loss among its population and has partnered with several non-profits that provide audiological testing and specialty care. One such entity is the Hear the World Foundation, a Swiss organization that provides audiological care and speech therapy to hearing-impaired children. Another gigantic effort to address and help those with hearing loss was the creation of the Haiti Deaf Academy, established by 160 deaf families after the 2010 earthquake in the small town of Leveque just outside the capital city of Port-a-Prince. The school carries out assessments, screening, and training of clinicians via volunteers from the Swiss company Sonova. Although this effort is working, the reality is that with the COVID-19 pandemic and in the event of a disaster wherein travel might be hampered or not possible, the use of Teleaudiology would allow the services provided by the Sonova volunteers to continue using the newly trained clinicians and technicians, who could be coached by the Sonova staff from their remote locations in Switzerland.[338]

No other pertinent data on the prevalence of hearing impairment or loss was found for the USVI and Haiti. Overall, the Teleaudiology services provide effortless accessibility to hearing specialists and services with many diverse options for a larger demographic population, especially those living in rural and remote areas, and thus would substantially benefit the nations of Africa, the USVI, and Haiti.

TELENURSING

African countries, USVI, and Haiti continue to face an unbalanced supply and availability of nurses and midwives' with this problem being exaggerated in rural, remote, and suburban areas where the population continues to experience substantial health inequalities.

The lack of a sufficient nursing workforce and health inequalities are not only caused by a persistent shortage of nurses but is also constrained by an unprecedented increase of out-migration and mobility of nurses to developed countries because of economic limitations, poor health policy, planning, and management. Furthermore, economic incentives or disincentives within the nursing community have not been reevaluated for several decades. As of today, the compensation incentive or remuneration is frequently described as being derisory and does not match with the current cost of living and therefore cannot decrease the gaps between private and public sector pay.

Healthcare specialties and subspecialty areas that treat age-related illnesses are affected by the burgeoning health demand and persistent shortage of healthcare providers. Therefore, the shortage coupled with the disparate dispersal of healthcare specialists across African countries, USVI, and Haiti are important issues that justify pressing attention and an alternative approach to nursing services delivery. Such an approach should move beyond the traditional delivery of healthcare service by decreasing persistent gaps and improving access to quality health services for most of the population.

Telenursing platforms are an exceptional approach that uses advanced technologies to enhance patient health and also have revealed huge advantages associated with diagnosis, consultation, and monitoring patients remotely from their home of residence through effective use of internet facilities such as computers, audio, and visual accessories and telephones. As with other telemedical specialties covered in this section, telenursing platforms are cost-effective and time-saving not only for nurses and midwives but also for patients preventing as travel is not needed to conduct the session. This approach can also be used for the provision of effective counseling and educational sessions through audio and video technology for healthcare providers, patients, and family members.

Overall, incorporating and implementing telenursing within the healthcare system will provide easy access to quality health specialties, improve the safety of patients and their health outcomes, increase workflow, and boost population satisfaction.

TELEPHARMACY

The pharmacy workforce remains not only insufficient, under-used, and undervalued but also pharmacists face difficulties performing their pharmaceutical care duties. An ongoing pharmacist workforce shortage coupled with a serious lack of clear, and long-term development strategies for recruitment and retention, has been affecting the production of pharmaceutical industry services.

The limited practicing pharmacists work either in public, private, or pharmaceutical industry sectors and are dispersed to the more urban localities leaving rural communities without access to pharmaceutical services, which often leads to the use of black-market enterprises and stand-up temporary pharmacies that may or may not be legitimate or may be staffed by persons without formal certified training, or with insufficient training. The few pharmacists that do work in remote areas work long hours incurring undue stress risking medication inaccuracies, misinterpretation of prescriptions and decreased motivation to remain in the field. Therefore, alternative approaches are required to sustain the capacity development of the pharmacist workforce to meet international standards related to pharmaceutical services and also ensure the provision of access to quality medicine.

Telepharmacy is not uncommon. Many pharmacies use Telepharmacy techniques and platforms by way of automated telephone-available medication refill services, text messaging to patients that prescriptions are ready for pick up, require refill order from a physician, and other services. Telepharmacy platforms have widely been accepted by many healthcare providers as it allows health services such as drug evaluation, patient therapy, and prescription verification by a distanced competent pharmacist for people living in rural and remote areas.

Furthermore, Telepharmacy is cost-effective, has economic benefits, is shown to have great patient satisfaction, and is helpful in augmenting pharmacy services wherein there is a scarcity of local pharmacists and pharmacy services; it is also timesaving for patients preventing travel over interminable distances to fill prescriptions in person.

The use of the platform appears to be a suitable alternative to the persistent workforce shortage and has proven to be an innovative way to offer access to effective quality pharmacy services to rural and regional localities.

CHAPTER FIVE:
TELEMEDICINE, POLITICS, AND REGULATIONS

POLITICAL AND ADMINISTRATIVE ENGAGEMENT

Political and administrative considerations are a key obstacle to adopting telemedicine services. These include challenges ranging from internal resistance to improve current regulatory policies and lack of interest, and concern of policymakers to provide sufficient funding to bring about effective infrastructure improvements. The existing condition of the healthcare industry requires effective regulatory and policy approaches that align with the true meaning and advantages of telemedicine services and the social and health needs of the population. Policy improvements in the health care industry will ensure the sustainable development of the effective implementation of telemedicine services and will formally regulate planning and funding process.

REINFORCING TELEMEDICINE PLATFORMS PROCEDURES

As shown in previous chapters, Telemedicine platforms are the future for African countries, the USVI, and Haiti's health care systems, mainly to improve provider communities' capacity to connect with the neglected remote and rural populations who have restrained access to quality healthcare specialists.

Lawmakers should reinforce and improve existing laws and regulations focusing on payment and coverage parity standards for telemedicine services, including patient agreement and rights, and privacy standards before being consulted or receiving any treatment from healthcare providers. The laws and regulations should provide a clear classification for telemedicine platforms which comprises store-and-forward technology, remote patient monitoring, teleconference, e-mail, and facsimile. In addition, laws and regulations should require all telemedicine services to be performed at the same level of quality of care as in-person consultation or treatment.

Lawmakers should formulate proper recommendations related to licensing, credentialing, and drug prescriptions through telemedicine platforms, including suggesting performance metrics to be implemented to measure the value of telemedicine services. Furthermore, the law and regulations should direct that payers such as public and private insurance organizations cover telemedicine services provided in place of an in-person appointment and satisfies the principles of care.

ALIGNING TELEMEDICINE POLICIES AND REGULATIONS

Telemedicine requires alignment of policies and regulations. A long-standing barrier to telemedicine services has been the existing laws regarding patient and provider relationships, along with medication-prescribing rules.

In some instances, a patient and provider relationship are designated as valid only after a face-to-face visit. However, with the approval and signature of the governing boards of African countries, the USVI, and Haiti, lawmakers could reformulate the definition of the provider-patient relationship to include telemedicine visits.

More telemedicine-friendly laws could also allow providers to prescribe controlled medications if needed, via telecommunications to pharmacies. Regulatory support for aligning telemedicine policies and regulations would also gather more support for private insurance agencies to develop policies that allow qualified public and private healthcare provider entities to bill for telemedicine/Telepharmacy services.

CHAPTER SIX:
LOOKING FORWARD: EMERGING RISKS

PART 1:
EMERGING TECHNOLOGICAL RISKS

Telemedicine has grown from simple cell phone conversations to multifaceted algorithmic-driven smartphone-based functions. As an emerging technology, telemedicine services foster effectiveness and accessibility, and its capacity of uninterrupted and instantaneous transmission of data over computer networks can come with a wide-ranging set of substantial risks. At every stage of the process, harmful acts can happen, including diagnostic failures, technical malfunctions, and confidentiality errors in patient self-show and security infractions. Also, many developers lack medical practice knowledge and do not include physicians in the mobile application and implementation growth, and this causes gaps, omissions, and errors in telehealth/;telemedicine development resulting in ineffective and/or difficult to navigate programs and processes. Further, they promote many of these applications to users with no proper security or performance assessment. [339]

Given these considerations, governments and healthcare providers must be knowledgeable of the probable emerging technological risks associated with practicing telemedicine services. Approaches to decrease emerging technology risks in telemedicine include:

1. People's protection awareness should pass through all stages of the telemedicine development life period.

2. Integrate protection assessment as part of practice and performance tests; such assessments must not be restricted to academic medical frameworks.

3. Apply the most recent data safety and encryption techniques to secure people's confidentiality.

4. Increase regulatory, expert, and healthcare organizations' engagement in establishing agreement-guided strategies, practical procedures, and rules, which must be renewed.

5. Complete publication of potential emerging technological risks before people register to use the telemedicine platforms.

6. Set up systems for healthcare providers and physicians to document telemedicine services and integrate them as part of daily work activities.

7. Increase attempts to reduce social risks by forming additional preventive measures for individuals and foreign-language speakers with moderate health knowledge.

The following security measures, among others, should be established and applied as well.

1. **Authentication:** Allows people to enter the system and access data through pathways such as log-in secret code, biometric scans, voice configuration, and smart identification card. Authentication procedures also let service administrators confirm certain users and their channels of the interface. Outside access must be restricted to those system networks that follow organizational safety measures.

2. **Patient/client identification:** Uses people integration profiles to promote correct verification at various locations. These profiles allow the cross-referencing of individual identifiers either from various domains or from a main consumer information server.

3. **Data control:** Ensures that an individual's data is stored and transferred in a classified way through the conception of a VPN, use of encryption technology, and/or file anonymization software. A rising quantity of medical practices also necessitates numerical signatures to confirm that data have not been changed by an unauthorized user. Encryption procedures similarly must broaden to stored data on portable devices or removable media, like laptop computers, tablets, smartphones, discs, and USB flash drives are an important source of data breaches.

4. **Data tracking:** Provides an assessment record of all interactions involving medical data, allowing the system authority to substantiate who has manipulated the system and/or retrieved consumer information.

Related monitoring technologies help recognize and shield against technical malfunctions and hacking.

5. **Protected access systems:** Protect telemedicine applications on wireless networks. It can exploit a range of safety mechanisms to offer both logical and physical restrictions, including firewalls and antivirus software that identifies malicious programs and activity.

In conclusion, telemedicine services are enhancing the health of people, especially those living in distant locations, and have the potential to transform health care delivery in the countries focused upon in this book.

The present increase in acceptance and incorporation into the workflow of healthcare systems, without uncertainty and diminishing reticence, will continue as the technology progresses and developments expand. Although certain telemedicine programs can avoid medical inaccuracies, emerging technological risks to individual protection are real. These risks need scholars, business organizations, and civil society representatives to focus on the role of telemedicine platforms in their countries. The major responsibility rests with governments and healthcare providers.

Governments and healthcare providers must evaluate the above risks in their country's framework and formulate corresponding guidelines and strategies, including social skills development and work assignment platforms, knowledgeable property and competition rules, and local technology adaptation and growth. They must balance their focus upon the moral confidence of accepting the technology-driven innovations in healthcare to improve access to quality and effectiveness. Adopting this approach should allow healthcare providers to conduct their practices comfortably using telemedicine technologies, thereby improving population safety and well-being.

PART 2:
EMERGING TECHNOLOGICAL RISKS: AVOIDING FRAUD SCHEMES

Although corruption in the healthcare industry is viewed as a global phenomenon, the consistent frequency of healthcare fraud in African countries, the USVI, and Haiti, however, is described as a serious, prevalent issue occurring at all levels, including in the healthcare delivery chain, with and between health care providers, members of staff, administrators, and providers of services.

Studies conducted by Thornton et al. (2015) reported that healthcare corruption happens frequently in the form of false/ phantom claims process, over-servicing, claiming for excluded products, coding irregularities, waiving of members deductibles, fragmenting billing codes, illegible service providers, double billing, kickbacks and self-referrals, and fraud risk management.[340]

The financial hardship of fraud, waste, ineffective and unenforced judicial monitoring policies, and mismanagement perpetrated daily costs billions, and increases insurance premiums; and also dispossesses African and Caribbean (US. Virgin Islands and Haiti) populations of accessible, affordable, quality healthcare services they deserve - especially those living in remote and rural localities.[341, 342]

Although corruption and bribery differ from country to country, as of today, there are still no exact data showing the scope of healthcare fraud in Africa and the Caribbean (US. Virgin Islands and Haiti). This lack of consequential data is because data mining techniques are not implemented in an efficacious manner, nor is the collection of such data a priority in Africa and Haiti. In. September 2020, the USVI held the first meeting of its Virgin Islands Health Care Fraud Task Force to address the primary form of healthcare fraud in the island-nation: Medicaid fraud wherein providers bill for services not rendered or bill higher codes.[343]

Transparency International, a prominent worldwide watchdog agency committed to exposing and stopping "corruption and promoting transparency, accountability, and integrity", indicated that it deems African countries among the world's most corrupt nations, an element contributing to the stunted growth and starvation of the African population. Further, several published articles, including the African Union study released in 2002, asserted that the constant bribery and gratifications are not only costing African countries more than $150 billion annually but also, approximately 75 million people in Sub-Saharan Africa are likely to have settled a payoff in the past year either to avert retaliation by law enforcement or courts or to access the fundamental social benefits that they lack.[344, 345]

While, in preceding years, the Latin America and Caribbean countries made fair steps in the fight against bribery and fraud, improvement against corruption in Haiti has not been achieved. In fact, corruption in Haiti is said to be endemic in all levels of government and public sector business as well. This never waning tide of corruption affects the healthcare system reinforcing the lack of preventive care, low spending on public health, continued incidences of preventable diseases such as cholera, and further visibly manifests itself throughout the nation's shoddy infrastructure. [346-348]

As of today, there are yet no significant policies or government objectives in place, focusing on the structural causes of corruption within the country. These features have earned the small island-nation the dubious title of most corrupt Caribbean nation by Transparency International. [349]

Corruption afflicts all aspects of life in many of Africa's nations, the USVI, and Haitian communities along with forming environments afflicted with structured crime systems, and money laundering, producing severe disruption of effective appropriation of resources for health services and other basic population needs.

One of the major challenges in successfully implementing and maintaining Telemedicine platforms in the USVI, Haiti, and Africa, will be the creation of mechanisms to monitor, eradicate, and punish fraud and corruption at all levels of government and in the public and private business sectors. In the absence of stringent laws that are readily enforced and upheld, corruption and fraud will continue to have deleterious impacts in all walks of life – not just health care, and telemedicine will be one more victim in a long line of failed programmatic efforts at improving access to equitable, quality, and accessible health care.

While it may be difficult to prevent all persistent fraud schemes, abuse, and well-funded cybersecurity attacks, many of today's fraud and abuses could be avoided by reinforcing current regulation and legislative laws to ensure better compliance in the practice of telemedicine platforms. Governments must foster political determination and show a continued long-term responsibility to anti-bribery reforms. Failing to enforce and mitigate telemedicine fraud, abuse, and cybersecurity schemes in a relationship with payment arrangements can provide a route to expensive repercussions.

Therefore, the development of this technology platform necessitates effective checks and balances via collaborative efforts of the government, healthcare providers, private sector, policymakers, regulators, and community members to form preventive measures against fraud and unsolicited expenses before they occur. Guidelines and advice, education, and compliance requirements, including professional liability policies, coverage, and legal counsel about the use of telemedicine platforms, demand to be established and enforced before healthcare providers use the technology.

Preventing fraud and misuse of telemedicine platforms requires strengthening anti-fraud beliefs that create avenues for deceitful actions and ensure all entities operating the telemedicine platforms have strong ethical principles and adopt good faith regulatory framework efforts to guarantee telemedicine services are delivered with integrity to the population in need.

Government enforcement agencies should readily and without restraint, enforce all regulations covering the use of telemedicine platforms, inclusive of mobile health, health information technology, and distant monitoring software used to provide needed services to the population. The different enforcement agencies must be at the front line of the improvement of international monitoring guidelines for health information technology and be deeply bonded in the regulatory efforts covering the telemedicine platform businesses.

A collaborative global framework with the World Health Organization (WHO) and the United Nations Office on Drugs and Crime (UNODC) can be formed through consultative assemblies to address international health fraud and stress the significance of reinforcing existing anti-fraud mechanisms in health policy and capacity building objectives.[350] This approach will offer a firm commitment to carry out cross-border, regional, and international strategies to identify and indict offenders following current domestic and regional legislations.

In summation, as the practice of telemedicine platforms continues to develop, the governments, healthcare providers, private sectors, policymakers, regulators, and community members using the technology services, should be not only mindful of the guidelines and legislations leading this rising industry, but also follow the corporate practice of medicine laws to avoid running afoul of fraud and misuse regulations when using telemedicine.

PART 3:
EMERGING HEALTH RISKS: NEW INFECTIOUS DISEASES AND HOW THEY MAY AFFECT OR LEAD TO CHANGES IN TELEMEDICINE

Since the World Health Organization (WHO) confirmed the novel Coronavirus (COVID-19) outbreak as a public health emergency of international concern, doubts are rising about the ability of African countries, the USVI, and Haiti to care for their populations in the midst of the rapidly expanding coronavirus pandemic.

As of March 2020, the Coronavirus (COVID-19) pandemic had impacted over 187 countries or territories, with more than 463,387 established infections and claimed higher than 20,912 deaths, according to the WHO. By December 2020, there were 77,793,186 confirmed cases of the virus: 1,710,967 reported deaths. [351] It is not untenable to proffer that in this scenario, telemedicine can be of immense benefit to health providers and patients – not only for those who may have COVID-19, but as importantly, for those in need of ongoing medical follow-up, and the diagnoses of other illnesses and conditions when travel to a medical facility is not possible or recommended due to disease spread.[352,353]

This COVID-19 outbreak has unveiled an unexplored frontier for telemedicine technologies. For years, people have pointed out telemedicine as an alternative to traditional public health services because it can lower costs, expand access to care, and can make doctors' work safer and more valuable. While developed countries such as the United States have embraced and endorsed the concept of using telemedicine technologies to protect healthcare providers and patients engaged in the reduction of COVID-19 infection rates. African countries, USVI, and Haiti governments are still behind in the use of the technology.

Presently, several of these countries are not only unable to take advantage of the untapped capacity of telemedicine services but are also not making this technology an important priority for providing high-quality care and minimizing exposure of infectious disease to healthcare providers and patients. Telemedicine technologies have been effective in protecting healthcare workers from harmful viruses such as Ebola outbreaks in the preceding years and are now showing promising results with COVID-19 by allowing remote consultations, examinations, and patient maintenance, resulting in diminishing human contact and protecting frontline employees.

Telemedicine technologies have not only grown into an alternate approach to provide care during this COVID-19 pandemic, but it has also helped keep sick individuals from gathering in hospital, urgent care, and clinic waiting rooms. From the assessment of an infected individual to the patterned delivery of therapy, telemedicine has been helping patients get the finest care, and the efficiency of consultation conducted by telemedicine is often the same compared to an in-person appointment. Healthcare providers can examine a remote patient located anywhere in the world, listen to the patient explain their symptoms, ask questions, and sense the same visual and hearing sensitivities as if the patient were face-to-face in the consultation room. Further, telemedicine systems also offer an opportunity for patients to interact with their family or loved ones in case they become quarantined, and the use is not constrained by geographic boundaries.

As African countries, USVI, and Haiti are fighting with the challenges of resolving the COVID-19 pandemic, the call for telemedicine technologies is obvious, and healthcare providers should work collaboratively with their authorities to remove obstacles restricting the whole practice of this great technology into the healthcare activities.

CHAPTER SEVEN:
FUTURE OF TELEMEDICINE

There is much to be passionate about regarding the prospect of the future of telemedicine technologies. With rapid innovation, it is reasonable that telemedicine platforms will become more widely adopted in the forthcoming years. As of now, technologies such as Google Glass and Apple Watch have been monitoring patients' health data and transferring it promptly to health providers.

Recognized applications, such as automatic robotic surgeries and the Digital Health Augmedix, have been providing dedicated clinical assistance and transforming clinician-patient conversation into medical documentation, so that healthcare specialist's emphasis on patient care issues is a patent illustration of the benefits of telemedicine.

In summation, telemedicine technology has a considerable role to play in the quality's improvement and effectiveness of health systems in African countries, the USVI, and Haiti, as it presents innovative avenues for interaction and partnership. However, to benefit from this technological break-through, the current constraints on telemedicine practice legislation, licensing provisions, and reimbursement policies must be corrected so that healthcare providers are rewarded, and patients are not paying exorbitant out-of-pocket fees. The fact is, telemedicine is a billion-dollar business, and its prospects are bright, and demand is expected to surmount these challenges.

The findings discussed here should help advance exploratory research procedures that will focus on major aspects of the successful implementation of telemedicine services and engender proposed actions to overcome related challenges.

CONCLUSION

Overall, this book has revealed there is substantial information about telemedicine technology and service, which, if acted upon, can assist in further strengthening healthcare systems, improve awareness, and cost-productivity in African countries, the USVI, and Haiti.

The ongoing deteriorating indicators of health in these countries call for a new look into the structure of current systems and an examination of innovative and resourceful ways to approach healthcare delivery and to re-structure delivery and systems to address continuing problematic courses of direction and related issues more thoroughly.

These nations must consider and face the fact that most of their populous are frightened about the shortage of specialists, the scarcity of medications, incorrect dosages and quantities at most health facilities, the terse and often unprofessional bedside manner of health employees, and the faulty and inept delivery of health services at many institutions, especially for the underprivileged, the elderly, the disabled, and those residing in rural and remote areas.

Some healthcare providers, partners, and community organizations recognize the benefits associated with telemedicine as it is attaining success in healthcare systems around the world. Telemedicine is no longer just a "nice-to-have" but is now a "must-have" for healthcare professionals and patients, especially for those living in remote areas during these doubtful times the COVID-19 pandemic has brought about.

A report by the Center for Disease Control and Prevention (CDC) asserted that people who live in rural areas are more likely than urban residents to die prematurely from the five leading causes of death: heart disease, cancer, unintentional injury, chronic lower respiratory disease, and stroke. An accurate statistic that is even more poignant during COVID-19.[354].

Telemedicine can help reduce obstacles to care for people who live far away from specialists or who have transportation or mobility issues. Instead of moving the patient to the clinical specialist, it is now commonplace and more conducive to use the power of technology to send the knowledge of the specialist right to the patient in need.

Ample evidence has shown that the safety and effectiveness of telemedicine can be achieved not only with the improvement of new collaborative work efforts between healthcare providers, stakeholders, and community members as joint problem solvers, but also by incorporating telemedicine within the health systems to allow the population to receive quality care and ease the burden of healthcare cost. This emphasizes the need for governments and healthcare authorities to issue or amend current Telemedicine Practice Guidelines to allow healthcare professionals the ability to provide healthcare services using telemedicine. Currently, there are no specific or singular legislation or statutory guidelines which deal with the practice of telemedicine in African countries, the USVI, and Haiti.

While each country crafts laws regulating the use and access of telemedicine, the legislative authorities should be more favorable to amend Telemedicine Practice Guidelines to allow cross-country consultations. National regulations are, by definition, confined to a country's geographic boundaries – i.e., applying only to that nation and its inhabitants. But telemedicine can be conducted without the limitation of physical and geographic boundaries, at least theoretically. Therefore, without more robust national frameworks for telemedicine, providers looking to offer cross-border services will be limited and could be exposed to the unauthorized (unlawful) practice of medicine.

Forming effective telemedicine financing policies will prevent the population from incurring tremendous out-of-pocket costs for healthcare services and ensure telemedicine is substantially funded to include continued functionality. This suggests that countries need adequate funding resources to cover the structural, organizational, and institutional factors impeding the implementation of telemedicine technologies. Implementing this technology lies in the hands of the governments, stakeholders, health professionals, and community organizations. However, it is recognized that healthcare executives consciously continue to exclude community representatives and healthcare providers who work in rural and remote localities from the decision-making processes. This exclusion prevents the sharing of compelling information and data about the local health situation and limits the desired (and needed) role of remote physicians and health practitioners as reliable partners in the delivery of health services.

Therefore, judicious collaborative efforts from all entities are needed and encouraged so that telemedicine services can provide necessary health solutions through direct clinical services, both intra- and inter-jurisdictional, training, and task shifting processes among health workers.

Achieving this at continental and national levels requires the determination of all entities, insight, coordination, and management of disparate factors. It must start with targeted identification of impediments to improvement along with honest, open discussions about those and the designation of collaborative efforts to remediate problems using technologies and cost-effective solutions sensitive to the reality of the poverty of those most in need.

Involving the population in the process will enhance access and acceptance. Innovative procedures for using resources and leveraging people's potential in the approaches illustrated in this book will contribute to reforming health system performance and provide solutions for the productive delivery of health services to the broadest population.

As the international health structural design undergoes transformation and wise spending is highlighted, the new strategic groundwork for the delivery of health services should encourage decision-making about innovations for enhanced health results without requiring enormous additional financial expenditure. Such a vision is possible to be achieved not only through technological approaches but also by the structured development of synergistic e-health strategy, incorporating telemedicine platforms at the national and international levels to guide public and private innovation and comprehensive user acceptance.

The expectation is that policymakers and healthcare leaders perceive the seriousness with which African countries, the USVI, and Haitian populations need innovations in their health systems.

RECOMMENDATIONS

The World Health Organization has been urging nations throughout the globe to consider long-range and lasting planned strategies for the development and implementation of telemedicine services. This book has unveiled a few of the recommendations that may, if acted upon, help strengthen healthcare systems, improve awareness, and provide cost-efficiency in African countries, the USVI, and Haiti.

The following are suggestions the governments of these countries must implement to successfully bring about widespread change in their existing healthcare systems through the addition of telemedicine technology:

1- Establish national and international telemedicine committees supported by ministries of health to offer advice on regulatory and strategy implementation, data safety measures, ethical concerns, interoperability, cultural and language matters, infrastructure, financial support, monitoring, and assessment.

2- Share policies with committing partners at all stages – from conception through implementation: community health specialists, academic establishments, health leaders, and policymakers.

3- Support and encourage telemedicine research and evaluation programs that embody procedures and approaches for knowledgeable interpretation.

4- Start simple — Healthcare facilities and other institutions should begin using telemedicine for simple services before gradually moving to complex use such as multi-provider calls. Telemedicine is tiered — Start with things easy to approach without additional technology, then proceed to higher levels of coordinated, multi-personnel services with augmented exam techniques.

5- Train providers — Training is a key component of a successful program; this will allow healthcare practitioners to become comfortable with the video and audio components and discuss any concerns.

6- Integrate telemedicine with other systems — Integrate telemedicine with other technologies such as electronic medical records to ensure efficiency and better data management. While integration could be challenging, benefits such as being able to quickly access population health information and having a single database for patient records makes the process meaningful and effective.

7- Establish reasonable expectations — Many telemedicine implementation programs struggled because of a lack of properly set objectives. Effective implementation is difficult without a project plan. Include all necessary steps from inception to completion and anticipate potential execution issues.

8- Consider the population and healthcare providers' knowledge related to the need for telemedicine implementation in the evaluation strategy formulation and practice in a broader structure of health improvements directed by clinical evidence and normative work.

9- Enhance the quality of deteriorating public health delivery through effective reorganization and telemedicine implementation that will improve healthcare facilities, drug distribution, and funding that provides universal health coverage and improves the population's well-being.

10- Expand the scope of telemedicine services to address, besides the general population, the needs of the vulnerable groups, such as the elderly and disabled populations.

11- Establish proper health financing procedures including, public health insurance, fiscal policy, and community financing.

12- Design health improvements that would be applied through innovative approaches of telemedicine, which can improve effective access to community health services, development, organization, and strategies.

13- Support the conducting of health service research and the sharing of public health best practices to promote and support telemedicine technologies and accelerate progress towards the achievement of national and internationally approved objectives of telemedicine platforms.

14- Analyze outcomes — Healthcare facilities and other institutions should track results from telemedicine after a period of service to find gaps in care, comparisons of health outcome from in-person physical visits to telemedicine coordinated visits, or opportunities to expand the resource. Health systems that implement this technology and these kinds of programs must examine what they are doing and create informative reports.

The bottom line is if the governments in African nations, Haiti and the

USVI are serious about providing their citizens with equitable access to a healthcare system that is fully functional then they must invite to the discussion and planning table with hospital administrators, financiers and concerned citizens. The goal must be to design a health care system that incorporates the true needs of the people. The planning must seriously consider and investigate viable funding options and designate them solely for the health system. Funding must also be specifically designated for and committed to programs of health education, equipment procurement and maintenance, and training in telemedicine. Universal Health Care must be a primary focus and be included in the early planning stages. A committee of knowledgeable and experienced subject matter experts must be brought in to conduct the research necessary to determine those medical specialties that would provide the most benefit via telemedicine platforms and enhancing infrastructure to support permanent stability of telemedicine platforms and the newly operable healthcare system. Without a committed and targeted approach, these countries will not turn the tide on the health system and health outcomes issues which have plagued them for years.

APPENDIX A:
TELEMEDICINE TERMINOLOGY

The following are some of the most common definitions and terms used in telemedicine.

Asynchronous: Sometimes, this term is used in describing the process of the store and forward transmission for sending information or medical images since the transmission takes place in one direction, as opposed to synchronous which, transmits in both directions.

Bandwidth: Measures a communications channel's information-carrying capacity; for a telemedicine service, this is a practical limit to its capabilities, cost, and size.

Bluetooth Wireless: Bluetooth refers to an industrial specification that applies to wireless area networks. Bluetooth technology offers a way of connecting and exchanging information between devices, including laptops, cell phones, PCs, video game consoles, digital cameras, and printers over an unlicensed and secure short-range radiofrequency.

Broadband: Communications (e.g., satellite, microwave, and broadcast television) with the ability to carry a wide range of various frequencies. It refers to signals being transmitted in a frequency-modulated manner over a portion of the total available bandwidth, which permits several messages to be transmitted simultaneously.

Clinical Information System: Relates to information about patient care, as opposed to administrative data. It is a hospital-based information system that has been designed for the collection and organization of data.

CODEC: This is an acronym for coder-decoder. It is a videoconferencing device (e.g., Panasonic, Sony, Tandberg, Polycom, etc.) which converts analog audio and video signals into audio and digital video code and vice versa. CODECs compress digital code to conserve a telecommunication path's bandwidth.

Compressed video: is the process of encoding a video file and sending it over a phone network, in such a way that it consumes less space than the original file and is easier to transmit over the network/Internet. It is a type of compression technique that reduces the size of video file formats by eliminating redundant and non-functional data from the original video file.

Computer-based Patient Record (CPR): Individual patient information in an electronic format that has provided access to accurate and complete patient information.

Consults: Primary care providers meet with or refer to medical specialists who may not be available locally.

Data Compression: A method used to reduce the volume of data. It is also used to reduce storage space requirements, bandwidth requirements, transmission times, and image processing. Some information loss takes place with some compression techniques, this might be clinically important or not, depending on the specific circumstances.

Diagnostic Equipment: (Cameras, Scope, and Other Types of Peripheral Devices): A hardware device separate from a central computer (e.g., camera, stethoscope, or digitizers) that can offer medical data input into a computer or accept output from one.

Medical Digital Camera: Imperx manufactures Industrial and Ruggedized CCD and CMOS cameras featuring high sensitivity and high dynamic range sensors for many Medical applications. With an easy to utilize, yet very powerful feature set, Imperx will help make any Medical imaging application a success. Some general uses for this kind of camera include wound care and dermatology. Healthcare providers can download the images produced onto a PC and then sent them over a network to a consultant or provider.

Digital Imaging and Communications in Medicine (DICOM): This is a communications standard for medical imaging devices. It is a set of protocols that are vendor-independent and describe how to identify and format images.

Distance Learning: The use of audio and video technologies allows students to attend training sessions and/or classes conducted from a remote location. Distance learning systems are interactive. They are a useful tool for delivering education and training to students that are widely dispersed, or sometimes, where an instructor cannot travel to the site where the students are located.

Distant Site: Refers to a telehealth site where a specialist or provider either consults with the patient or sees the patient from a distant or remote location other than in-person face-to-face interaction. Other common names used for this term include referral site, physician site, provider site, specialty site, consulting site, and hub site.

Document Camera: This camera can display type or written information (e.g., lab results), graphics (e.g., ECG strips), photographs, and X-rays sometimes.

Electronic Data Interchange (EDI): receive and send data between two trading partners without human invention or paper.

Electronic Patient Record: Individual patient information in an electronic format that provides access to accurate and complete patient data, links to medical information, clinical decision support systems, reminders, alerts, and other types of aids.

Encryption: A system for encoding data on an email or web page where only the computer system or person allowed to access the information can retrieve and decode it.

Firewall: Computer software and hardware that blocks unauthorized communications between external networks and an organization's or individual's computer network.

Full-motion Video in medical setting: A full-motion **video** (FMV) is the rapid display of a series of images by a computer in such a way that the person viewing it perceives fluid movement. An FMV can consist of live action, animation, computer-generated imagery, or a combination of those formats. It typically includes sound and can include text superimposed over the **video**.

Guideline: A procedure or policy statement for determining a course of action or providing guidance on setting standards.

Health Education Video conferencing allows health care professionals to conduct continuing education programs with attendees in multiple locations. Patients can use these technologies to take disease management courses or receive other important health information.

Home Health Care and Remote Monitoring Systems: Care that is provided via distanced technology to patients and their families in their residences to promote, maintain, or restore health; or to minimize the effects of illness and disability, including terminal illnesses.

Informatics: Using information technologies and computer science to process and manage knowledge, information, and data.

Integrated Services Digital Network (ISDN): A common dial-up transmission path used for videoconferencing. ISDN services are on-demand services where another IDSN based device is dialed, and per-minute charges are accumulated at a certain contracted rate.

Interactive (two-way) Audio-Video Technology: Live Video (synchronous) is a two-way interaction between a person (patient, caregiver, or provider) and a provider using audiovisual telecommunications technology. This type of service is also referred to as "real-time" and may serve as a substitute for an in-person encounter when such not available.

Live video can be used for consultative, diagnostic, and treatment services. Video devices can include videoconferencing units, peripheral cameras, videoscopes, or web cameras, computer monitors, plasma/LED TV, LCD projectors, and even tablet computers. Remote ICU monitoring programs at hospitals provide 24-hour backup, supervision, and support to ICU medical staff by utilizing a combination of real-time video to observe patients, interactive video communications with on-site ICU providers, and digital patient monitoring equipment.

Interactive Television/Video: Video conferencing technologies that make possible for synchronous, two-way interactive audio and video signals to be transmitted for delivering distance education, telemedicine, or telehealth services. The acronyms are often used to refer to VTC (video teleconference), IATV, or ITV.

Internet Protocol (IP): The protocol for sending data from one computer over the internet to another. Every computer connected to the Internet has at least one IP address that identifies it from all the other computers using the Internet.

Interoperability: This refers to two or more systems (software, networks, communication devices, computers, and other types of information technology components) being able to interact with each other and exchange information so that healthcare providers can achieve predictable results. There are three different interoperability types: technical, clinical, and human/operational.

ISDN Basic Rate Interface (BRI): is an Integrated Services Digital Network

(ISDN) configuration intended primarily for use in subscriber lines similar to those that have long been used for voice-grade telephone service. As such, an ISDN BRI connection can use the existing telephone infrastructure at a business. An ISDN interface can also provide 128K of bandwidth used for videoconferencing as well as simultaneous data and voice services. A multiplexer can link multiple BRI lines for higher bandwidth levels to be achieved.

ISDN Primary Rate Interface (PRI): An ISDN interface standard that operates using one 64K data channel and 23 64K channels. When the correct multiplexing equipment is used, the user can select the IDN PRI channels for a video call.

JCAHO: This is an acronym for the Joint Commission on Accreditation of Healthcare Organizations. This organization evaluates standards of quality in service, patient outcomes, the provision of health care accreditation, improvement of safety, and quality in health services provided to the public by health services organizations.

Lossless: This is a data compression that allows users to reconstruct images without losing the information from the original copies. It can achieve a compression ratio of 2:1 for images with color.

Lossy: This is a compressing data process with a high ratio. During the process healthcare providers could remove unnecessary information when reconstructing patient images.

Mobile Telehealth Clinic: is a vehicles such as a van, trailer, or any mobile unit which allows patients to take advantage of receiving high quality healthcare services closer to their home. The services are administered by health care professionals. This is helpful to those who live in locations distant from a hospital. Some mobile units are equipped with medical technologies that are found in the hospital, like mobile CT, MRI, and Tele Dentistry.

Mobile Health Technology (mHealth): Mobile health or mHealth, a relatively new and rapidly developing aspect of technology-enabled health care, is the provision of health care services and personal health data via mobile devices, such as cell phones, tablet computers, and PDAs. mHealth often includes the use of dedicated application software (apps), which are downloaded onto devices. Applications can range from targeted text messages that promote healthy behavior to wide-scale alerts about disease outbreaks, to name a few examples. South Central Telehealth Resource Center video on mHealth exemplifies many of the most popular forms and uses of mHealth mobile applications.

Modalities for Telemedicine

Four main modalities used: **(https://www.cchpca.org/about/about-telehealth)**
- Interactive audio-video technology (a.k.a. live video).
- Store-and-forward technology.
- Remote patient monitoring technology.
- Mobile health technology.

Multiplexer shortened or **MUX:** is a combinational logic circuit designed to switch one of several input lines through to a single common output line by the application of a control signal.

Multi-point Control Unit or MCU: This is a device used to connect a few videoconferencing sites into a single system. Healthcare providers also refer to Multipoint Control Unit as the "bridge".

Multipoint Teleconferencing: This is the process of connecting multiple users from different sites. It allows electronic communication between the users as well as transmissions of video, voice, and data between computers. Multipoint teleconferencing requires the use of a multipoint control unit or a bridge to connect different sites for the videoconference.

Network Integrators: These are organizations that give services and develop software to allow the sharing of data, videos and voices, and communication between different devices and systems.

Originating Site: This is where the patient and physician are located during the time of consultation. This site is also called a patient site, remote site, spoke site, or rural site. The site allows patients to access their personal health information from any location with the help of the Internet.

Patient Exam Cameras: These cameras are used to examine the patient's overall condition. The different types of patient exam cameras are handheld cameras, camcorders, gooseneck cameras, and those which may be placed above the set-top units. Analog and digital cameras are available, and the ones that should be used depend on the connection to the set-top unit.

Peripheral Device: This is a device that can be connected to the computer. Examples of peripheral devices include mouse pointers, keyboards, video cameras, scanners, and monitors used for clinics and hospitals, including weight scales and pulse oximeters.

Presenters or Patient Presenters: They are the individuals who provide telehealth services and examine patients. Such presenters should be in the medical field (physicians, registered nurses, and licensed practical nurses), and they must have experience in providing health services to patients.

Telepharmacy Solutions: This refers to the provision of pharmacy services to patients using communication technology and electronic information. Healthcare providers use this when patients cannot avail themselves of such services in person.

Regional Health Information Organization/Health Information Exchange (RHIO/HIE): These are organizations that ensure the quality, efficiency, and safety of the health services delivered by Telehealth.

Remote Patient Monitoring (RPM) Technology: Remote patient monitoring (RPM) uses digital technologies to collect medical and other forms of health data from individuals in one location and electronically send that information securely to health care providers in a different location for assessment and recommendations. This service allows a provider to continue to track healthcare data for a patient once released to home or a care facility, reducing readmission rates.

Router: This is a device that provides connections to at least two networks in an organization. It provides network connections in multiple locations, and it finds the best route between two sites. It tells the videoconferencing devices where the destination devices can be found, and it will find the best way to gather the information from that specific destination.

Standard: This term refers to the benchmark used to measure the quality of the results. The standard is established by the overseeing, accountability, or certifying authority to make sure that organizations are achieving the desired results.

Store and Forward: This is a form of telemedicine consultation which allows for the electronic transmission of medical information, such as digital images, documents, and pre-recorded videos through secure email communication. Transmission of recorded health history (for example, pre-recorded videos and digital images such as x-rays and photos) through a secure electronic communications system to a practitioner, usually a specialist who uses the information to evaluate the case or render a service outside of a real-time or live interaction. As compared to a real-time visit, this service provides access to data after healthcare providers have collected it and involves communication tools such as secure email.

Store-and-Forward Technology: Store-and-forward technologies allow for the electronic transmission of medical information, such as digital images, documents, and pre-recorded videos, through secure email communication. Store-and-forward technologies are most used in radiology, pathology, dermatology, and ophthalmology: Transmission of recorded health history (for example, pre-recorded videos and digital images such as x-rays and photos) through a secure electronic communications system to a practitioner, usually a specialist who uses the information to evaluate the case or render a service outside of a real-time or live interaction. As compared to a real-time visit, this service provides access to data after it has been collected and involves communication tools such as secure email.

Switch: In the videoconferencing world, switch refers to the device responsible for selecting the path that will be used in transmitting the video.

Synchronous: This term refers to the interactive connections between two videos when the information is transmitted at the same time for both directions.

Systems Integration: This involves bringing together two systems and devices and sharing data and information between the two systems.

T1/DS1: This is a service for telephone lines that provide a bandwidth data service of 1.544 Mbps.

T3/DS3: This is a carrier that allows the users to have a bandwidth data service of up to 45 Mbps. Transmission Control Protocol/Internet Protocol–This involves the standard rules for establishing and maintaining network conversation between two computers with the help of the Internet.

Task shifting: Implies the rational redistribution of tasks among health workforce teams. Specific tasks are moved, where appropriate, from highly qualified health workers to health workers who have fewer qualifications to make more efficient use of the available HRH.

Telecare: Telecare refers to technology that allows consumers to stay safe and independent in their own homes. For example, Telecare may include consumer-oriented health and fitness apps, sensors, and tools that connect consumers with family members or other caregivers, exercise tracking tools, digital medication reminder systems, or early warning and detection technologies.

Telecommunications Providers: These are the entities allowed by the governments to provide telecommunications services to all residents and institutions.

Telemedicine: Defined as the use of telecommunications technologies to support the delivery of all kinds of medical, diagnostic, and treatment-related services by doctors. For example, this includes conducting diagnostic tests, closely monitoring patient progress after treatment or therapy, and facilitating access between health care providers and patients who are in different physical locations.

Telemedicine/Telehealth: These two terms are used to describe the use of technology and telecommunications to exchange medical information from one place to another to improve the patient's health status. Telemedicine is sometimes involved in direct patient clinical services, which include diagnosis and treatment of patients.

Telehealth: Telehealth is like Telemedicine but includes a wider variety of remote healthcare services beyond the doctor-patient relationship. It often involves services provided by nurses, pharmacists, or social workers, for example, who help with patient health education, social support and medication adherence, and troubleshooting health issues for patients and their caregivers.

Teleconferencing: This is the interaction between multiple users across various sites with the use of interactive electronic communication. This involves the transfer of video and audio through computer and video systems. This interaction is usually live and is used in the diagnosis or monitoring of patient in-home care.

Telementoring: is the use of video, audio, and other electronic and telecommunication processing technologies to offer individual guidance. A good example of this would be a physician mentoring a local healthcare provider new in the healthcare industry.

Telemonitoring: this is the process of using video, audio, and other electronic and telecommunication systems to transfer live information between computers to monitor the health status of a patient from a distance. A good example would be home care.

Telematics: The integration or use of information processing that is based on a computer and using telecommunications to allow programs and data transfer between computers.

Telepresence: The use of robotics and other technologies to allow a medical practitioner to perform a procedure at a certain location by using devices and receiving sensory information or feedback, which contributes to a sense of presence and allowing certain achievement in a procedure.

Teleradiology: The transfer of radiological images. X-rays, MRIs, and CTs are many radiological images. Healthcare providers use these images for consultation, diagnosis, or interpretation.

Universal Service Administrative Company: Abbreviated as USAC, the Universal Service Administrative Company administers USFs, or Universal Service Funds to allow easy access to telecommunication services across the country.

Ultrasound Device: This is any device that uses high-frequency sound technology to examine internal body organs. These devices are used to detect tumors and other inner body organ abnormalities.

Wi-Fi: Wi-Fi is a family of wireless network protocols, based on the IEEE 802.11 family of standards, which are commonly used for local area networking of devices and Internet access. Wi-Fi is a trademark of the non-profit Wi-Fi Alliance, which restricts the use of the term Wi-Fi Certified to products that successfully complete interoperability certification testing.

Videoconferencing Systems: This equipment and software allows real-time two-way communication, which is usually in the form of digitized audio and video. Healthcare providers use these systems for meetings without having to be in the same room. Video conferencing can provide cost-effective access to care for patients who are institutionalized or incarcerated. Video conferencing has historically been the most common application of Telemedicine/Telehealth care use and is an effective consultation tool for several applications, including Emergency Room / Intensive Care Unit support, and could connect emergency providers with medical specialists who otherwise would not be available for consults.

APPENDIX B:
REFERENCES

[1] https://www.who.int/csr/resources/publications/introduction/en/index1.html

[2] https://www.moh.gov.jm/infectious-diseases-remain-a-major-threat-to-the-caribbean-region/

[3] Gubler, D. J. (1998). Resurgent Vector-Borne Diseases as a Global Health Problem. *Emerging Infectious Diseases,* 4(3), 442-450. https://dx.doi.org/10.3201/eid0403.980326; Actually, retrieved from https://wwwnc.cdc.gov/eid/article/4/3/98-0326_article

[4] https://www.mckinsey.com/industries/healthcare-systems-and-services/our-insights/strengthening-sub-saharan-africas-health-systems-a-practical-approach

[5] Callwood, G. B.; Campbell, D.; Gary, F.; et al. (2012. Health and Health

Care in the U. S. Virgin Islands: Challenges and Perceptions. Retrieved from: https://www.ncbi.nlm.nih.gov/pmc/articles/PMC3573759/pdf/nihms370925.pdf

[6] https://www.priviahealth.com/blog/what-can-independent-providers-learn-from-health-centers/

[7] Delamater, P.L., Messina, J.P., Shortridge, A.M. et al. Measuring geographic access to health care: raster and network-based methods. Int J Health Geogr 11, 15 (2012). https://doi.org/10.1186/1476-072X-11-15. Retrieved from https://ij-healthgeographics.biomedcentral.com/articles/10.1186/1476-072X-11-15

[8] Access to Primary Care. Retrieved from https://www.healthypeople.gov/2020/topics-objectives/topic/social-determinants-health/interventions-resources/access-to-primary

[9] Healthcare in the Remote Developing World: Why healthcare is inaccessible and strategies towards improving current healthcare models. Retrieved from http://www.hhpronline.org/articles/2016/11/10/healthcare-in-the-remote-developing-world-why-healthcare-is-inaccessible-and-strategies-towards-improving-current-healthcare-models

[10] https://bphc.hrsa.gov/about/what-is-a-health-center/index.html

[11] A Universal Truth: No Health Without a Workforce Third Global Forum on Human Resources for Health Report (2015). Retrieved from https://www.who.int/workforcealliance/knowledge/resources/

GHWA_AUniversalTruthReport.pdf

[12] https://www.who.int/workforcealliance/knowledge/resources/hrhreport2013/en/

[13] World bank org/curated/en/755121468137986975/International-Finance-Corporation-IFC-annual-report-2007-creating-opportunity. Retrieved from http://documents1.worldbank.org/curated/en/755121468137986975/pdf/41234optmzd0PA10071English01PUBLIC1.pdf

[14] https://qz.com/520230/africa-has-about-one-doctor-for-every-5000-people/

[15] https://foreignpolicy.com/2010/06/11/countries-without-doctors/

[16] https://www.who.int/workforcealliance/knowledge/resources/GHWA-a_universal_truth_report.pdf

[17] http://www1.umn.edu/humanrts/crc/togo2005b.html.

[18] United Nations World mortality report 2013 [Internet] New York (NY): UN; 2013; Retrieved from https://www.un.org/en/development/desa/population/publications/pdf/mortality/WMR2013/World_Mortality_2013_Report.pdf

[19] http://www.un.org/en/development/desa/population/publications/pdf/mortality/WMR2013/World_Mortality_2013_Report.pdf

[20] Deaton, A. S., & Tortora, R. (2015). People in sub-Saharan Africa rate their health and health care among the lowest in the world. Health affairs (Project Hope), 34(3), 519–527. https://doi.org/10.1377/hlthaff.2014.0798. Retrieved from https://www.ncbi.nlm.nih.gov/pmc/articles/PMC5674528/

[21] (2004). MDG 6: Combat HIV/AIDS, Malaria and Other Diseases. Retrieved from: https://www.who.int/topics/millennium_development_goals/diseases/en/

[22] Infant Mortality Rate by Country. Retrieved from: https://www.worldatlas.com/articles/countries-with-the-highest-infant-mortality-rates.html.

[23] A Redefining Moment for Africa. Retrieved from: https://www.transparency.org/news/feature/a_redefining_moment_for_africa

[24] Corruption. Retrieved from: https://www.globalsecurity.org/military/world/haiti/corruption.htm

[25] Virgin Islands News – Crime and Corruption Updates. Retrieved from: http://claudettevferron.com/virgin-islands-news-crime-and-corruption-updates

[26] Agbenorku, P. (2012). Corruption in Ghanaian Healthcare System: The Consequences. Journal of Medicine and Medical Sciences, Vol. 3(10) pp.622-630, October 2012. Retrieved from: www. Transparency. Org/content/download/4912/28857/file /Ghanaian_Chronicle_06-02-02.pdf

[27] Clausen, L. B. (2015). Taking on the Challenges of Health Care in Africa. Retrieved from: https://www.gsb.stanford.edu/insights/taking-challenges-health-care-africa

[28] Infectious Diseases Remain a Major Threat to the Caribbean Region. Retrieved from: https://www.moh.gov.jm/infectious-diseases-remain-a-major-threat-to-the-caribbean-region

[29] Redmond, H. Haiti and Health Care: Poverty, Profit, and Disease. https://plenty.org/haiti-and-health-care/

[30] Institut Haïtien de l'Enfance (Haiti); ICF International. Évaluation de pre-station des services de soins de santé, Haïti, 2013. Rockville, MD: IHE / ICF International. Retrieved from https://www.dhsprogram.com/pubs/pdf/SR211/SR211.pdf

[31] Evaluation de la Prestation des Services de Soins de Sante 2013. Retrieved from http://mspp.gouv.ht/site/downloads/EPSSS.pdf

[32] Ministère de la Santé Publique et de la Population (Haiti). Bilan 5 ans du MSPP Octobre 2011–February 2016. Port-au-Prince: MSPP; 2016. Retrieved from https://issuu.com/alexandrefritzarios/docs/bilan_5_ans_du_mspp_web

[33] Ekine,S. (2013). Cholera and Healthcare in Haiti. Retrieved from: https://www.pambazuka.org/food-health/cholera-and-health-care-haiti#:~:text=One%20medical%20improvement%20to%20HUEH%20and%20which%20is,cared%20for%20over%201%2C000%20

patients%20TB%20since%202010.

[34] Haiti's Struggling Healthcare System. Retrieved from: https://new-int.org/blog/2013/02/25/haiti-healthcare.

[35] Haiti: New World Bank Report Calls for Increased Health Budget and Better Spending to Save Lives (2017). Retrieved from: https://www.worldbank.org/en/news/press-release/2017/06/26/haiti-new-world-bank-report-calls-for-increased-health-budget-and-better-spending-to-save-lives

[36] https://www.marketplace.org/2017/06/16/for-many-haitians-street-dispensaries-are-only-source-medicine/

[37] Health Program in Haiti: Clinics and Dispensaries. Retrieved from: https://www.asase.org/en/prog_haiti_sante.php

[38] Better Spending, Better Care: A Look at Haiti's Health Financing. Retrieved from: https://www.worldbank.org/en/country/haiti/publication/better-spending-better-care-a-look-at-haitis-health-financing

[39] Better Spending, Better Care: A Look at Haiti's Health Financing: A Summary Report (English). Retrieved from: http://documents.worldbank.org/curated/en/393291498246075986/summary-report

[40] Haiti: New World Bank Report Calls for Increased Health Budget and Better Spending to Save Lives. Retrieved from: https://www.worldbank.org/en/news/press-release/2017/06/26/

haiti-new-world-bank-report-calls-for-increased-health-budget-and-better-spending-to-save-lives

[41] https://www.worldbank.org/en/news/press-release/2017/06/26/haiti-new-world-bank-report-calls-for-increased-health-budget-and-better-spending-to-save-lives.

[42] Better Spending, Better Care: A Look at Haiti's Financing. Retrieved from: https://www.scribd.com/document/430204214/116682-WP-v1-Wb-Haiti-English-PUBLIC-Summary

[43] Haitian President to US: Send Aid to Haiti Gov't Not NGOs. (2014). VOA News. Retrieved from: https://www.voanews.com/americas/haitian-president-us-send-aid-haiti-govt-not-ngos

[44] https://www.worldbank.org/en/news/press-release/2017/06/26/haiti-new-world-bank-report-calls-for-increased-health-budget-and-better-spending-to-save-lives

[45] Corruption. Retrieved from: https://www.globalsecurity.org/military/world/haiti/corruption.htm.

[46] The Undermining of Haitian Health Care: Setting the Stage for Disaster. Retrieved from: https://nacla.org/news/undermining-haitian-health-care-setting-stage-disaster.

[47] Haiti – Heath: Nearly 40% of Haitian Doctors Settle Abroad. Retrieved from: https://www.haitilibre.com/en/

news-21951-haiti-health-nearly-40-of-haitian-doctors-settle-abroad.html

[48] Young, N., (2017). Haiti's Troubled Healthcare System. Retrieved from: https://nonprofitquarterly.org/haitis-troubled-healthcare-system/

[49] Global Corruption Barometer: Latin America and the Caribbean 2019 – Citizens' Views and Opinions of Corruption. Retrieved from: https://www.transparency.org/whatwedo/publication/global_corruption_barometer_latin_america_and_the_caribbean_2019

[50] Chattopadhyay, S. (2013). Corruption in Healthcare and Medicine: Why Should Physicians and Bioethicists Care and What Should They do? Indian Journal of Medical Ethics, Vol. 10, No. 3 (2013). Retrieved from: http://ijme.in/articles/corruption-in-healthcare-and-medicine-why-should-physicians-and-bioethicists-care-and-what-should-they-do/?galley=html

[51] Global Corruption Barometer: Latin America and the Caribbean 2019 – Citizens' Views and Opinions of Corruption. Retrieved from: https://www.transparency.org/whatwedo/publication/global_corruption_barometer_latin_america_and_the_caribbean_2019

[52] https://www.worldometers.info/world-population/united-states-virgin-islands-population

[53] https://2020census.gov/en/conducting-the-count/island-areas/virgin-islands.html

[54] https://countrymeters.info/en/United_States_Virgin_Islands

[55] Community Needs Assessment: Understanding the Needs of vulnerable Children and Families in the U. S. Virgin Islands Post Hurricanes Irma and Maria. Retrieved from: https://cfvi.net/wp-content/uploads/2019/03/CFVI-CERC-Community-Needs-Assessment-E-Report_February-2019_Bookmarked.pdf

[56] https://stcroixsource.com/2019/11/06/report-hundreds-may-have-died-due-to-storm-damage-to-v-i-health-system/

[57] https://www.buzzfeednews.com/article/briannasacks/us-virgin-islands-hospitals

[58] https://www.npr.org/2018/02/04/582256476/in-the-u-s-virgin-islands-health-care-remains-in-a-critical-state

[59] World Off Track in Meeting 2030 Agenda, UN Deputy Chief Warns, Calls for Solidarity in COVID-19 Recovery. Retrieved from: https://news.un.org/en/story/2020/07/1068551

[60] Universal Health Coverage (UHC). Retrieved from: https://www.who.int/news-room/fact-sheets/detail/universal-health-coverage-(uhc)

[61] World Health Organization Blames Africa's Health Care Inequality on Lack of Political Will. Retrieved from: https://www.dw.com/en/world-health-organization-blames-africas-health-care-inequality-on-lack-of-political-will/a-40283418

[62]   Berki, S. E. (1986). A Look at Catastrophic Medical Expenses and the Poor. Retrieved from https://www.healthaffairs.org/doi/10.1377/hlthaff.5.4.138

[63]   Galbraith, A. A.; Wong, S. T.; Kim, S.E.; Newacheck, P. W. (2005). Out-of-Pocket Financial Burden for Low-Income Families with Children: Socioeconomic Disparities and Effects of Insurance. Health Serv Res. 2005 Dec.; 40(6 Pt 1): 1722-1736. Doi: 10.1111/j.1475-6773.2004.00421.x Retrieved from: https://www.ncbi.nlm.nih.gov/pmc/articles/PMC1361224/

[64]   While Poverty in Africa Declined, Number of Poor Has Increased. Retrieved from: www.worldbank.org/en/region/afr/publication/poverty-rising-africa-poverty-report.

[65]   U. S. Foundation: Funding for Africa, 2015 Edition Retrieved from: http://foundationcenter.org/gainknowledge/research/pdf/funding_for_africa2015.pdf

[66]   Wealth Gap Widening for More than 70% of Global Population, Researchers Find. Retrieved from: https://www.theguardian.com/global-development/2020/jan/22/wealth-gap-widening-for-more-than-70-per-cent-of-global-population-researchers-find#:~:text=The%20income%20gap%20has%20been,a%20world%20without%20global%20warming.

[67]   Inequality – Bridging the Divide. Retrieved from: https://www.un.org/en/un75/inequality-bridging-divide

[68]   https://www.oxfam.org/en/5-shocking-facts-about-extreme-global-inequality-and-how-even-it

[69]   https://www.dw.com/en/world-health-organization-blames-africas-health-care-inequality-on-lack-of-political-will/a-40283418

[70]   African Hospitals Not Built for African Presidents – Why African Presidents Get Treated Abroad. Retrieved from: https://www.africanexponent.com/post/9174-african-presidents-love-seeking-treatment-abroad

[71]   https://www.dw.com/en/world-health-organization-blames-africas-health-care-inequality-on-lack-of-political-will/a-40283418

[72]   Legitimating Inequality: Fooling Most of the People All of the Time. Retrieved from: https://www.researchgate.net/publication/46467781_Legitimating_Inequality_Fooling_Most_of_the_People_All_of_the_Time.

[73]   John Thompson 1991. Ideology and Modern Culture, Stanford: Stanford University Press

[74]   Accelerating Poverty Reduction in Africa: In Five Charts. Retrieved from: https://www.worldbank.org/en/region/afr/publication/accelerating-poverty-reduction-in-africa-in-five-charts.

[75]   Quiet Corruption' Impedes African Development, World Bank Report(2010. Retrieved from https://www.kff.org/news-summary/quiet-corruption-impedes-african-development-world-bank-report-says/

[76] Africa Development Indicators 2010: Silent and Lethal – How Quiet Corruption Undermines Africa's Development. Retrieved from: https://documents.worldbank.org/pt/publication/documents-reports/documentdetail/485121468192847343/africa-development-indicators-2010-silent-and-lethal-how-quiet-corruption-undermines-africas-

[77] 'Quiet Corruption' Impedes African Development World Bank Says. Retrieved from: https://khn.org/morning-breakout/gh-031610-world-bank-report/

[78] https://www.who.int/health_financing/topics/financial-protection/en/

[79] Transparency International, Global Corruption Report. London and Ann Arbor; 2006. Retrieved from: https://images.transparencycdn.org/images/2006_GCR_HealthSector_EN.pdf

[80] Robinson M. Foreword and Executive Summary. Transparency International, Global Corruption Report. London and Ann Arbor; 2006

[81] Vian T. Corruption and the Health Care Sector. Sectoral Perspectives on Corruption. USAID, Washington; 2002. Retrieved from: https://bmcinthealthhumrights.biomedcentral.com/articles/10.1186/1472-698X-12-5

[82] Kohler J. Fighting Corruption in the Health Sector: Methods. Tools and Good Practices, United Nations Development Programmes; 2011. Retrieved from: https://www.who.int/bulletin/volumes/96/9/18-209502/en/

[83]	Corruption in Global Health: The Open Secret. Retrieved from: https://www.thelancet.com/journals/lancet/article/PIIS0140-6736(19)32527-9/fulltext?hss_channel=tw-27013292

[84]	Vian T. Corruption and the Health Care Sector. Sectoral Perspectives on Corruption. USAID, Washington; 2002. Retrieved from: https://bmcinthealthhumrights.biomedcentral.com/articles/10.1186/1472-698X-12-5

[85]	Kaufmann, Daniel, Aart C. Kraay, and Massimo Mastruzzi (2007). "Governance Matters VI: Aggregate and Individual Governance Indicators 1996–2006." World Bank Policy Research Working Paper 4280, Washington, DC: World Bank. Retrieved from http://info.worldbank.org/governance/wgi/pdf/WGI.pdf

[86]	The Global Constitution. Retrieved from: http://globalcommunitywebnet.com/GlobalConst/DRAFT5.HTM

[87]	Health Systems Governance. Retrieved from: https://www.who.int/healthsystems/topics/stewardship/en/.

[88]	Eshetu, E. B., & Woldesenbet, S. A. (2011). Are there particular social determinants of health for the world's poorest countries? African health sciences, 11(1), 108–115. Retrieved from: https://www.ncbi.nlm.nih.gov/pmc/articles/PMC3092326/.

[89]	Marmot M, Friel S, Bell R, Houweling TA, Taylor S; Commission on Social Determinants of Health. Closing the gap in a generation: health equity through action on the social determinants of health. Lancet.

2008 Nov 8;372(9650):1661-9. doi: 10.1016/S0140-6736(08)61690-6. PMID: 18994664.

[90] Marmot M, Friel S, Bell R, Houweling TA, Taylor S; Commission on Social Determinants of Health. Closing the gap in a generation: health equity through action on the social determinants of health. Lancet. 2008 Nov 8;372(9650):1661-9. doi: 10.1016/S0140-6736(08)61690-6. PMID: 18994664. Retrieved from: https://www.ncbi.nlm.nih.gov/pmc/articles/PMC3092326.

[91] Marc H, Byong-Joon K, editors. Building Good Governance: Reforms in Seoul. National Center for Public Productivity; 2002.

[92] Barro R. Democracy and Growth. Journal of Economic Growth. 1996;1:1–27.

[93] Petersen I, Marais D, Abdulmalik J, et al. Strengthening mental health system governance in six low-and middle-income countries in Africa and South Asia: challenges, needs, and potential strategies. Health Policy Plan. 2017;32(5):699–709. doi:10.1093/heapol/czx014. Retrieved from https://academic.oup.com/heapol/article/32/5/699/3090698

[94] Marais DL, Petersen I. Health system governance to support integrated mental health care in South Africa: challenges and opportunities. Int J Ment Health Syst. 2015;9(1):14. doi:10.1186/s13033-015-0004-z

[95] World Mortality 201 Retrieved from https://www.un.org/en/development/desa/population/publications/pdf/mortality/

World-Mortality-2017-Data-Booklet.pdf.

[96]   Under Five Mortality: Retrieved from: https://data.unicef.org/topic/child-survival/under-five-mortality/

[97]   Health Systems in Africa: Community Perceptions and Perspectives. Retrieved from: https://www.afro.who.int/sites/default/files/2017-06/english---health_systems_in_africa---2012.pdf

[98]   Haiti's Troubled Healthcare System. Retrieved from: https://nonprofitquarterly.org/haitis-troubled-healthcare-system/

[99]   In the U.S. Virgin Islands, Health Care Remains in a Critical State. Retrieved from: https://www.npr.org/2018/02/04/582256476/in-the-u-s-virgin-islands-health-care-remains-in-a-critical-state

[100] 3 Ways to Improve Healthcare in Africa. Retrieved from: https://www.weforum.org/agenda/2015/01/3-ways-to-improve-healthcare-in-africa.

[101] https://www.usaid.gov/haiti/global-health.

[102] World Bank. World Development Indicators (2006). Retrieved from https://documents.worldbank.org/en/publication/documents-reports/documentdetail/918311468316164759/world-development-indicators-2006

[103] Growing Threat from Counterfeit Medicines. Retrieved from: https://

www.who.int/bulletin/volumes/88/4/10-020410/en/

[104] 1 in 10 Medical Products in Developing Countries is Substandard or Falsified. Retrieved from: www.who.int/en/news-room/detail/28-11-2017-1-in-10-medical-products-in-developing-countries-is-substandard-or-falsified

[105] Counterfeit Drugs in Africa: current Situation, Causes and Countermeasures. Retrieved from: https://inventa.com/en/news/article/545/counterfeiting-of-fake-drugs-in-africa-current-situation-causes-and-countermeasures

[106] Up to 30% of All Medicines in Africa are Fake. Retrieved from: https://www.health24.com/Medical-schemes/News/Up-to-30-of-all-medicines-in-Africa-are-fake-20140619.

[107] Triple Burden: Disease in Developing Nations. Retrieved from: https://www.researchgate.net/publication/285088034_The_triple_burden_Disease_in_developing_nations/link/5720e73a08aeaced7890726b/download

[108] http://www.healthdata.org/research-article/global-age-sex-specific-fertility-mortality-healthy-life-expectancy-hale-and

[109] Global Health. Retrieved from: https://ourworldindata.org/health-meta

[110] World Bank and WHO: Half the World Lacks Access to Essential Health Services, 100 Million Still Pushed into Extreme Poverty Because

of Health Expenses. Retrieved from: https://www.who.int/news/item/13-12-2017-world-bank-and-who-half-the-world-lacks-access-to-essential-health-services-100-million-still-pushed-into-extreme-poverty-because-of-health-expenses

[111] How is Poverty Related to Access to Care and Preventive Healthcare? Retrieved from: https://poverty.ucdavis.edu/faq/how-poverty-related-access-care-and-preventive-healthcare

[112] Mapp: "in the Virgin Islands, We've Long Had Universal Healthcare." Retrieved from: https://sottvi.news/mapp-universal-healthcare/

[113] What Health Reform Means to the American Territories. Retrieved from: https://www.theatlantic.com/politics/archive/2017/08/what-health-reform-means-to-the-american-territories/538056/

[114] Islands of Progress: The Caribbean's Journey to Universal Health Coverage. Retrieved from: https://assets.kpmg/content/dam/kpmg/tt/pdf/2018-UHC-Caribbean-TL-Final.pdf

[115] Telemedicine: Opportunities and Developments in Member States. Report on the Second Global Survey on eHealth. Global Observatory for eHealth Series – Volume 2. Retrieved from: https://www.who.int/goe/publications/goe_telemedicine_2010.pdf

[116] Schulte, A.; Majerol, M; & Nadler, J. (2019). Narrowing the Rural-Urban Health Divide: Bringing Virtual Health to Rural Communities. https://www2.deloitte.com/us/en/insights/industry/public-sector/

virtual-health-telemedicine-rural-areas.html

[117] Digitization Continues: Bryan Convenes Workgroup Focused on Implementing Telehealth Services in USVI. (2020). Retrieved from: https://viconsortium.com/vi-government/virgin-islands-digitization-continues-bryan-convenes-workgroup-focused-on-implementing-telehealth-services-in-usvi

[118] Plesson Pioneers Telehealth in the USVI (2020). Retrieved from: http://www.virginislandsdailynews.com/business/plessen-pioneers-telemedicine-in-the-usvi/article_343b3a0f-fa1d-5baa-9ade-34c1280c3048.html

[119] Governor Bryan Announces 'Healthier Horizons' Initiative, Sweeping Healthcare Reform for the U. S. Virgin Islands. Retrieved from: https://www.vi.gov/healthier-horizons/

[120] Telemedicine: Opportunities and Developments in Member States. Report on the Second Global Survey on eHealth. Global Observatory for eHealth Series – Volume 2. Retrieved from: https://www.who.int/goe/publications/goe_telemedicine_2010.pdf

[121] What is the Difference Between Telemedicine and Telehealth? Retrieved from: https://blog.cureatr.com/whats-the-difference-between-telemedicine-and-telehealth#:~:text=While%20telemedicine%20refers%20specifically%20to%20remote%20clinical%20services%2C,continuing%20medical%20education%2C%20in%20addition%20to%20clinical%20services.%22

[122] WHO. A health telematics policy in support of WHO's Health-For-All strategy for global health development: report of the WHO group consultation on health telematics, 11–16 December, Geneva, 1997. Geneva, World Health Organization, 1998.

[123] Exploring the History of Telemedicine (& the Future). Retrieved from: https://save.health/telemedicine-3/history

[124] A Brief History of Telemedicine. Retrieved from: https://www.electronicdesign.com/technologies/components/article/21770508/a-brief-history-of-telemedicine

[125] Strehle, E. M.; Shabde, N. One Hundred Years of Telemedicine: Does This New Technology Have a Place in Pediatrics? Retrieved from: https://www.ncbi.nlm.nih.gov/pmc/articles/PMC2082971/pdf/956.pdf

[126] Craig, John & Patterson, Victor. (2005). Introduction to the Practice of Telemedicine. *Journal of Telemedicine and Telecare*. 11. 3-9. 10.1258/1357633053430494. Retrieved from: https://www.researchgate.net/publication/7908096_Introduction_to_the_practice_of_telemedicine

[127] Currell R et al. Telemedicine versus face-to-face patient care: effects on professional practice and health care outcomes. *Cochrane Database of Systematic Reviews*, 2000, Issue 2.

[128] Wooten, R.; Jebamani, L. S.; Dow, S. A. E-Health, and the Universitas 21 Organization: 2. Telemedicine and Underserved Populations.

Retrieved from: http://archive.u21health.org/sites/u21health.org/files/ehealth_and_U21_2.pdf

[129]   https://searchnetworking.techtarget.com/definition/asynchronous.

[130]   Difference Between Synchronous vs Asynchronous Transmission. Retrieved from> https://techdifferences.com/difference-between-synchronous-and-asynchronous-transmission.html

[131]   Global Estimates: Life Expectancy and Leading Causes of Death. Retrieved from: https://www.who.int/gho/mortality_burden_disease/life_tables/situation_trends/en/(2)https://data.worldbank.org/indicator/

[132]   https://howafrica.com/a-look-at-the-list-of-african-and-caribbean-countries-with-a-high-life-expectancy/

[133]   Ranking the Caribbean by Life Expectancy. Retrieved from: http://curacaochronicle.com/region/ranking-the-caribbean-by-life-expectancy

[134]   Lainscak M, Blue L, Clark AL, Dahlström U, Dickstein K, et al. (2011). Self-care management of heart failure: practical recommendations from the Patient Care Committee of the Heart Failure Association of the European Society of Cardiology. Eur J Heart Fail. 2011 Feb;13(2):115-26. doi: 10.1093/eurjhf/hfq219. Epub 2010 Dec 10. PMID: 21148593. Retrieved from: https://onlinelibrary.wiley.com/doi/full/10.1093/eurjhf/hfq219

[135] Inglis SC, Clark RA, Dierckx R, et al. Structured telephone support or non-invasive telemonitoring for patients with heart failure. Retrieved from: https://heart.bmj.com/content/103/4/255

[136] Khunlertkit A, Carayon P. Contributions of tele-intensive care unit (Tele-ICU) technology to quality of care and patient safety. J Crit Care. 2013 Jun;28(3):315.e1-12. doi: 10.1016/j.jcrc.2012.10.005. Epub 2012 Nov 14. PMID: 23159139.

[137] Study: Telemedicine Reduces Pediatric Medication Errors. Retrieved from: https://www.davisenterprise.com/news/local/ucd/study-telemedicine-reduces-pediatric-medication-errors/

[138] Dharmar M, Kuppermann N, Romano PS, Yang NH, Nesbitt TS, Phan J, Nguyen C, Parsapour K, Marcin JP. Telemedicine consultations and medication errors in rural emergency departments. Pediatrics. 2013 Dec;132(6):1090-7. doi: 10.1542/peds.2013-1374. Epub 2013 Nov 25. PMID: 24276844.

[139] Crafton, D. (2014). Telepharmacy Services Increasingly Filling Rural Need: Remote Medication Review Said to Help Reduce Medication Errors. Retrieved from: https://www.spokanejournal.com/local-news/telepharmacy-services-increasingly-filling-rural-need/

[140] Meidl, Tracy & Woller, Thomas & Iglar, Arlene & Brierton, Dennis. (2008). Implementation of pharmacy services in a telemedicine intensive care unit. American journal of health-system pharmacy : AJHP : official journal of the American Society of Health-System Pharmacists.

65. 1464-9. 10.2146/ajhp070682.

[141]   Telehealth in Rural Communities. Retrieved from: https://www.cdc.gov/chronicdisease/resources/publications/factsheets/telehealth-in-rural-communities.htm.

[142]   Healthcare and Economic Growth in Africa, The United Nations Economic commission for Africa (UNECA), New York, 27 September 2018. Retrieved from: http://gbchealth.org/wp-content/uploads/2018/09/PPT_27Sept2018-FINAL_22092018-4.pdf

[143]   World Health Organization. The Declaration of Alma-Ata: The International Conference on Primary Health Care, Alma-Ata, USSR, 6–12 September 1978. WHO: Copenhagen; 2000. Retrieved from: https://www.who.int/publications/almaata_declaration_en.pdf

[144]   Health for All Rural People: The Durban Declaration. Adopted at the 2nd World Rural Health Congress.

[145]   Health for All Rural People: The Durban Declaration. Adopted at the 2nd World Rural Health Congress. Retrieved from: https://www.sbmfc.org.br/wp-content/uploads/media/file/GT%20Medicina%20Rural/durban%20declaration.pdf

[146]   Patterson V et al. Supporting hospital doctors in the Middle East by email telemedicine: something the industrialized world can do to help. *Journal of Medical Internet Research*, 2007, 9(4):e30. Retrieved from: https://www.swinfencharitabletrust.org/publications/

academic-papers/062_J+Med+Internet+Res+2007+-+9+(4)+e+30.pdf

[147] Johnston, K. (2004). The cost-effectiveness of technology transfer using telemedicine. Health Policy and Planning. 19. 302-309. 10.1093/heapol/czh035.

[148] Mukundan S II et al. Trial telemedicine system for supporting medical students on elective in the developing world. *Academic Radiology*, 2003, 10(7):794-797.

[149] Sozen C, Kisa A, Kavuncubasi S. Can rural telemedicine help to solve the health care access problems in Turkey? *Clinical Research and Regulatory Affairs*, 2003, 20(1):117-126.

[150] Martinez A et al. Analysis of information and communication needs in rural primary health care in developing countries. *IEEE Transactions on Information Technology in Biomedicine*, 2005, 9(1):66-72.

[151] Pradhan MR. ICTs application for better health in Nepal. *Kathmandu University Medical Journal*, 2004, 2(2):157-163.

[152] Wootton R. Telemedicine and developing countries – successful implementation will require a shared approach. *Journal of Telemedicine and Telecare*, 2001, 7(Suppl. 1): S1-S6/

[153] Wootton R. Design and implementation of an automatic message-routing system for low-cost telemedicine. *Journal of Telemedicine and Telecare*, 2003, 9(Suppl. 1): S44-S47.

[154] Alverson DC et al. Transforming systems of care for children in the global community. *Pediatric Annal*, 2009, 38(10):579–585

[155] Lee S et al. The role of low-bandwidth telemedicine in surgical pre-screening. *Journal of Pediatric Surgery*, 2003, 38(9):1281–1283.

[156] Kifle M, Mbarika V, Datta P. Telemedicine in sub-Saharan Africa: The case of teleophthalmology and eye care in Ethiopia. *Journal of the American Society for Information Science & Technology*, 2006, 57(10):1383–1393.

[157] Wootton R, Menzies J, Ferguson P. Follow-up data for patients managed by store and forward telemedicine in developing countries. *Journal of Telemedicine and Telecare*, 2009, 15(2):83–88./

[158] Kifle M, Mbarika V, Datta P. Telemedicine in sub-Saharan Africa: The case of teleophthalmology and eye care in Ethiopia. *Journal of the American Society for Information Science & Technology*, 2006, 57(10):1383–1393./

[159] Kiviat AD et al. HIV online provider education (HOPE): The Internet as a tool for training in HIV medicine. *The Journal of Infectious Diseases*, 2007, 196(Suppl. 3): S512–S515.

[160] New Telemedicine Strategies Help Hospitals Address COVID-19. Retrieved from: www.modernhealthcare.com/patients/new-telemedicine-strategies-help-hospitals-address-covid-19

[161] Yaghobian S, Ohannessian R, Mathieu-Fritz A, Moulin T. National survey of telemedicine education and training in medical schools

in France. Journal of Telemedicine and Telecare. 2020;26(5):303-308. doi:10.1177/1357633X18820374

[162] FDA and CDC Promote Telemedicine During COVID-19 Outbreak. Retrieved from: www.mmm-online.com/home/channel/regulatory/fda-and-cdc-promote-telemedicine-during-covid-19-outbreak

[163] Moltu C, Stefansen J, Svisdahl M, Veseth M. Negotiating the coresearcher mandate - service users' experiences of doing collaborative research on mental health. Retrieved from https://www.researchgate.net/publication/236146080_How_to_Enhance_the_Quality_of_Mental_Health_Research_Service_Users'_Experiences_of_Their_Potential_Contributions_Through_Collaborative_Methods. (click on 'read full text).

[164] https://raccoongang.com/blog/difference-between-formal-and-informal-learning/

[165] www.igi-global.com/dictionary/technology-enhanced-learning-continuing-medical.

[166] Mirza, M., Kratz, M., Medeiros, D., Pina, J., Richards, J., Zhang, X., Fraser, H., Bailey, C., & Krishnamurthy, R. (2012). Building the foundations of an informatics agenda for global health - 2011 workshop report. Online journal of public health informatics, 4(1), ojphi.v4i1.4027. https://doi.org/10.5210/ojphi.v4i1.4027. Retrieved from https://www.ncbi.nlm.nih.gov/pmc/articles/PMC3615805/#:~:text=The%20 2005%2058th%20World%20Health%20Assembly%20eHealth%20

Resolution,effective%20practices%2C%20policies%2C%20and%20 standards%20in%20eHealth.%20a

[167] WHA58.25 eHealth Summary. Retrieved from: https://www.who.int/ healthacademy/media/WHA58-28-en.pdf?ua=1

[168] World Health Organization eHealth – Report by the Secretariat. Retrieved from: https://www.who.int/healthacademy/media/en/ eHealth_EB-en.pdf?ua=1

[169] Hendler, Shadbolt, Hall, Berners-Lee, and Weitzner 2008. Web Science: An Interdisciplinary Approach to Understanding the Web. Retrieved from: https://dl.acm.org/doi/fullHtml/10.1145/1364782.1364798

[170] Hebda TL, Czar P. (2002). *Handbook of Informatics for Nurses & Healthcare Professionals.* 4th ed. Upper Saddle River, NJ: Pearson Prentice Hall; 2009. https://doi.org/10.1016/j.aorn.2009.06.016.

[171] Andrews V. Using telemedicine in clinical decision-making. *Practice Nursing.* 2014. Published Online:18 Feb 2014 https://doi.org/10.12968/ pnur.2014.25.1.42

[172] Demiris, George PhD; Oliver, Debra Parker PhD; Courtney, Karen L. MSN, RN Ethical Considerations for the Utilization of Telehealth Technologies in Home and Hospice Care by the Nursing Profession, Nursing Administration Quarterly: January-March 2006 - Volume 30 - Issue 1 - p 56-66

[173]   https://www.afro.who.int/health-topics/ageing.

[174]   Social Security: Virgin Islands QuickFacts. Retrieved from: https://assets.aarp.org/rgcenter/econ/ss_facts_05_vi.pdf.

[175]   https://countrymeters.info/en/United_States_Virgin_Islands#facts.

[176]   https://www.who.int/countries/hti/en/.

[177]   Moore, Z.; Angel, D.; Bjerregaard, J., et al. (2017). eHealth in Wound Care: From Conception to Implementation; Published Online:18 Dec 2017https://doi.org/10.12968/jowc.2015.24.Sup5.S1. Retrieved from: https://www.magonlinelibrary.com/doi/abs/10.12968/jowc.2015.24.Sup5.S1

[178]   https://www.healthit.gov/topic/health-it-health-care-settings/telemedicine-and-telehealth

[179]   (2020) Chen, Edward T.; Improving Patient Care with Telemedicine Technology; from Impacts of Information Technology on Patient Care and Empowerment. Retrieved from https://www.igi-global.com/chapter/improving-patient-care-with-telemedicine-technology/235949

[180]   Gulube SM, Wynchank S. Telemedicine in South Africa: Success or failure? Journal of Telemedicine and Telecare. 2001;7(2_suppl):47-49. doi:10.1258/1357633011937100.

[181] Corr P. (1998). Teleradiology in KwaZulu-Natal. A pilot projects. S Afr Med J. 1998;88 (1):48–9. Retrieved from: https://www.ajol.info/index.php/samj/article/view/148681

[182] Wamala, D. S., & Augustine, K. (2013). A meta-analysis of telemedicine success in Africa. Journal of pathology informatics, 4, 6. https://doi.org/10.4103/2153-3539.112686. Retrieved from https://www.ncbi.nlm.nih.gov/pmc/articles/PMC3709418/

[183] Africa Telemedicine Outlook and Opportunities. Retrieved from: https://www.reportlinker.com/p04887125/Africa-Telemedicine-Outlook-andOpportunities.html).

[184] Ten years After the Information Society Summit, the General Assembly Examines Progress and Challenges Related to Digital Boom. Retrieved from: https://www.un.org/press/fr/2015/ag11741.doc.htm

[185] Adeyinka MB. Fundamentals of modern telemedicine in Africa. Inf Med. 1997;36:95–8; retrieved from https://www.ncbi.nlm.nih.gov/pmc/articles.

[186] Pan African e-network Project. Inauguration of Pan-African e-network Project (Phase 2) TCIL Bhawan, New Delhi on 16 th August 2010. Retrieved from: https://www.mea.gov.in/press-releases.htm?dtl/912/Inauguration+of+2nd+phase+of+PanAfrican+eNetwork+Project+by+EAM

[187] Faculte de Medicine de Pharmacie et d'Odonto Stomatologie,

Mali(FMPOS). http://fmos.usttb.edu.ml/

[188] Havranek, E. G.; Sharfi,A.R.; et al (2011). Low-cost Telemedicine. Khartoum-Sudan. BJUI Vol 107.Issue 11 June 2011; pp.1701-1702 https://doi.org/10.1111/j.1464-410X.2011.10229.x

[189] Nzeyimana D. (2012) Assessment of telemedicine in Rwanda, current and future State. Retrieved from https://www.ghdonline.org/tech/discussion/assessment-of-telemedicine-in-rwanda-current-and-f/

[190] Jambusaria A. The Advantages of telemedicine. Retrieved from https://telemedicine.tripod.com/advantages.htm

[191] Elbel, M. St. John's is Territory Trailblazer for Telemedicine. Published in St. John Tradewinds, A Community Newspaper. September 21- October 4,2009.Retrieved from https://ufdcimages.uflib.ufl.edu/UF/00/09/39/99/00069/00009-21-2009.pdf

[192] McCann, E. (2012). Haiti After the Quake: Telehealth Helps Heal One of the World's Poorest Countries. Retrieved from https://www.healthcareitnews.com/news/haiti-after-quake-telehealth-helps-heal-one-worlds-poorest-countries

[193] https://www.hrw.org/world-report/2019/country-chapters/haiti

[194] Padgett, T. (2015). Telemedicine for Haiti: The University of Miami Makes Trauma More Survivable https://www.wlrn.org/post/telemedicine-haiti-university-miami-makes-trauma-more-survivable#stream/.

[195]   Telemedicine in Haiti ... A Humble Assessment of Where We Are. (2010). Retrieved from http://medtechiq.ning.com/profiles/blogs/telemedicine-in-haiti-a

[196]   Telemedicine at Hospital Scre Couer. Retrieved from http://crudem.org/telemedicine-at-hopital-sacre-coeur/

[197]   Haiti Politics. Retrieved from https://www.globalsecurity.org/military/world/haiti/politics.htm

[198]   Marta Hurtado, "Press Briefing Note on Haiti Unrest," Office of the U.N. High Commissioner for Human Rights, November 1, 2019. Retrieved from https://www.ohchr.org/EN/NewsEvents/Pages/DisplayNews.aspx?NewsID=25247

[199]   World Health Organization Regional Office for Africa, 2013. Retrieved from https://www.afro.who.int/publications/work-who-african-region-2012-2013-biennial-report-regional-director

[200]   Shunned from Bond Market, U. S. Virgin Islands Faces Cash Crisis; Retrieved from: https://www.reuters.com/article/us-usa-virginislands-crisis-idUSKBN1AI0D2

[201]   State of Health Financing in Africa. The World Health Organization 2013. Retrieved from https://www.afro.who.int/sites/default/files/2017-06/state-of-health-financing-afro.pdf.

[202]   WHO. (2003) Abuja Declaration. African summit on Roll Back Malaria.

Geneva: WHO/Roll Back Malaria Partnership. Retrieved from: https://apps.who.int/iris/handle/10665/66391

[203] WHO. (2008f) Closing the gap in health equity through action on the social determinants of health. Geneva: World Health Organization Commission on Social Determinants on Health. Retrieved from http://www.who.int/ social determinants/thecommission/finalreport/ en/index.html) accessed 25/10/2011.

[204] Jennett PA, Affleck Hall L, Hailey D, Ohinmaa A, Anderson C, Thomas R, Young B, Lorenzetti D, Scott RE. The socio-economic impact of telehealth: a systematic review. J Telemed Telecare. 2003;9(6):311-20. doi: 10.1258/135763303771005207. PMID: 14680514. Retrieved from https://pubmed.ncbi.nlm.nih.gov/20696073/

[205] 5 Ways Telemedicine is Helping Rural Hospitals & Their communities. Retrieved from https://relymd.com/blog-5-ways-telemedicine-is-helping-rural-hospitals/

[206] Graham LE, Zimmerman M, Vassallo DJ, et al. Telemedicine--the way ahead for medicine in the developing world. Trop Doct. 2003;33:36-8.

[207] Ganapathy K. Telemedicine and neurosciences in developing countries. Surg Neurol. 2002 Dec;58(6):388-94. doi: 10.1016/s0090-3019(02)00924-2. PMID: 12517618.

[208] Oberholzer M, Christen H, Haroske G, et al. Modern telepathology: a distributed system with open standards. Curr Probl

Dermatol. 2003;32:102–14. Available at https://books.google.com/books?hl=en&lr=&id=F2gyQlDgptgC&oi=fnd&pg=PA102&dq=Oberholzer+M,+Christen+H,+Haroske+G,+et+al.+Modern+telepathology:+a+distributed+system+with+open+standards.+Curr+Probl+Dermatol.+2003%3B32:102%E2%80%9314&ots=a-kW0ir1Nr&sig=6nrI16kBVCoQ4BdsqYE2R-nht28#v=onepage&q&f=false

[209] Wright D. Telemedicine and developing countries. A report of study group 2 of the ITU Development Sector. J Telemed Telecare. 1998;4(Suppl 2):1–85.

[210] Craig J, Patterson V. Introduction to the practice of telemedicine. *Journal of Telemedicine and Telecare*, 2005. Retrieved from https://www.researchgate.net/publication/7908096_Introduction_to_the_practice_of_telemedicine

[211] Currell R et al. Telemedicine versus face-to-face patient care: effects on professional practice and health care outcomes. Cochrane Database of Systematic Reviews, 2000, Issue 2. https://doi.org/10.1002/14651858.CD002098

[212] Strehle EM, Shabde N. One hundred years of telemedicine: does this new technology have a place in paediatrics? Archives of Disease in Childhood 2006;91:956-959.

[213] Arn H. Eliasson, MC USA, Ronald K. Poropatich, MC USA, Performance Improvement in Telemedicine: The Essential Elements, Military Medicine, Volume 163, Issue 8, August 1998, Pages 530–535, https://

doi.org/10.1093/milmed/163.8.530; actually, retrieved from https://academic.oup.com/milmed/article/163/8/530/4831942

[214] World health report 2010 - Health systems financing: the path to universal coverage. Geneva: World Health Organization; 2010. Retrieved from https://www.who.int/whr/2010/en/

[215] The impact of health insurance in Africa and Asia: a systematic review .Retrieved from https://www.who.int/bulletin/volumes/90/9/12-102301/en/

[216] https://www.transparency.org/topic/detail/health.

[217] *Quiet Corruption' Impedes African Development, World Bank Report Says.* Retrieved from https://www.kff.org/news-summary/quiet-corruption-impedes-african-development-world-bank-report-says/

[218] How does corruption affect health care systems, and how can regulation tackle it? https://www.euro.who.int/en/data-and-evidence/evidence-informed-policy-making/publications/hen-summaries-of-network-members-reports/how-does-corruption-affect-health-care-systems,-and-how-can-regulation-tackle-it#:~:text=Corrupt%20activity%20is%20likely%20to%20damage%20the%20ability,deteriorate%2C%20especially%20among%20the%20most%20vulnerable%20population%20groups.

[219] Eikelboom, Robert H. (2012) *The Telegraph and the Beginnings of Telemedicine in Australia.* Retrieved from https://www.researchgate.net/

publication/233384000_The_telegraph_and_the_beginnings_of_telemedicine_in_Australia

[220] Mbarika, Victor W.A. & Okoli, Chitu (2003), *Telemedicine in Sub-Sharan Afrrica: A Proposed Delphi Study (2003)*. Retrieved from https://www.researchgate.net/publication/221183561_Telemedicine_in_Sub-Saharan_Africa_A_Proposed_Delphi_Study

[221] Mbarika, Victor W.A. & Okoli, Chitu (2003), *Telemedicine in Sub-Sharan Afrrica: A Proposed Delphi Study (2003)*. Retrieved from https://www.researchgate.net/publication/221183561_Telemedicine_in_Sub-Saharan_Africa_A_Proposed_Delphi_Study

[222] Project of Telemedicine Collaboration in Healthcare in Senegal. Available at https://www.researchgate.net/publication/281897680_Project_of_telemedicine_for_collaboration_in_healthcare_in_Senegal

[223] https://borgenproject.org/poverty-in-the-virgin-islands/#:~:text=A%20 2010%20U.S.%20census%20found%20that%2022%20percent,poverty%20 level%20were%20families%20led%20by%20single%20mothers.

[224] https://sottvi.news/trouble-in-paradise-the-ever-growing-cost-of-living-in-the-virgin-islands/

[225] Forecasting the global shortage of physicians: an economic- and needs-based approach. Retrieved https://www.who.int/bulletin/volumes/86/7/07-046474/en/

[226] Fonn, Ray & Blaauw 2011). Fonn S., Ray S. & Blaauw D, 2011, 'Innovation to improve health care providers and health systems in sub-Saharan Africa – Promoting agency in mid-level workers and district managers', Global Public Health. Retrieved from: https://www.researchgate.net/publication/44804493_Innovation_to_improve_health_care_provision_and_health_systems_in_sub-Saharan_Africa_-_Promoting_agency_in_mid-level_workers_and_district_managers

[227] Heath, S. Understanding Physician Shortage Issues, Patient Care Access. Retrieved from https://patientengagementhit.com/news/understanding-physician-shortage-issues-patient-care-access

[228] Forecasting the global shortage of physicians: an economic- and needs-based approach https://www.who.int/bulletin/volumes/86/7/07-046474/en/

[229] The health worker shortage in Africa: are enough physicians and nurses being trained? Retrieved from https://www.who.int/bulletin/volumes/87/3/08-051599/en/

[230] Diagnosing Africa's Medical Brain Drain. Retrieved from https://www.un.org/africarenewal/magazine/december-2016-march-2017/diagnosing-africa%E2%80%99s-medical-brain-drain

[231] https://www.reuters.com/article/us-african-doctors-migration-idUSTRE7AO00O20111125

[232] Aluttis, Christoph, Tewabech Bishaw, and Martina W. Frank. 2014.

"The Workforce for Health in a Globalized Context – Global Shortages and International Migration." *Global Health Action.* https://doi.org/10.3402/gha.v7.23611. Retrieved from https://doi.org/10.3402/gha.v7.23611

[233] https://ysjournal.com/the-critical-shortage-of-healthcare-workers-in-sub-saharan-africa-a-comprehensive review.

[234] https://ysjournal.com/the-critical-shortage-of-healthcare-workers-in-sub-saharan-africa-a-comprehensive review.

[235] https://www.worldatlas.com/articles/the-countries-with-the-fewest-doctors-in-the-world.html.

[236] https://mo.ibrahim.foundation/news/2018/brain-drain-bane-africas-potential

[237] Causes and Effects of Brain Drain in Nigeria. Retrieved from https://researchcyber.com/causes-effects-brain-drain-nigeria/

[238] African Brain Drain: Is There an Alternative. Retrieved from https://en.unesco.org/courier/january-march-2018/african-brain-drain-there-alternative

[239] The Global Tug-of-War for Health Care Workers. Retrieved from https://www.migrationpolicy.org/article/global-tug-war-health-care-workers/

[240] Social and Economic Determinants of Health. Retrieved from https://www.afro.who.int/health-topics/social-and-economic-determinants-health

[241] How Social and Economic Factors Affect Health. Retrieved from http://www.publichealth.lacounty.gov/epi/docs/SocialD_Final_Web.pdf

[242] https://telradsol.com/benefits-of-teleradiology/

[243] https://dcmsys.com/2019/09/29/advantages-of-teleradiology/

[244] https://realrads.com/2020/02/27/8-benefits-of-teleradiology/

[245] https://www.psychiatry.org/patients-families/what-is-telepsychiatry

[246] https://www.sinclairmethod.org/top-5-benefits-telepsychiatry/

[247] https://psychsolutions.com/benefits-of-telepsychiatry/

[248] https://specialistdirectinc.com/telecardiology-articles/uncategorized/7-benefits-of-telecardiology-for-critical-access-hospitals/

[249] https://specialistdirectinc.com/telecardiology-articles/uncategorized/how-telecardiology-services-can-benefit-rural-communities/

[250] Mocumbi AO, Ferreira MB. Neglected cardiovascular diseases in Africa: challenges and opportunities. JAm Coll Cardiol 2010;55:680-7. Retrieved from https://www.jacc.org/doi/10.1016/j.jacc.2009.09.041

[251] Mocumbi A. O. (2012). Lack of focus on cardiovascular disease in sub-Saharan Africa. Cardiovascular diagnosis and therapy, 2(1), 74–77. https://doi.org/10.3978/j.issn.2223-3652.2012.01.03. Retrieved from https://www.ncbi.nlm.nih.gov/pmc/articles/PMC3839174/

[252] Antony KK. (1980). The pattern of cardiac failure in Northern Savanna Nigeria. Trop Geogr Med 1980;32:118-25.

[253] Oyoo GO, Ogola EN. Clinical and socio demographic aspects of congestive heart failure patients at Kenyatta National Hospital, Nairobi. East Afr Med J. 1999 Jan;76(1):23-7. PMID: 10442143.

[254] Shiel, Jr., William C. Asthma Rates Increasing . . . Are Environmental Exposures? Retrieved from https://medicinenet.com/asthma_rates_increasing/views.htm

[255] WHO Regional Committee for Africa. Cardiovascular diseases in the African region: current situation and perspectives-report of the regional director 2005. Retrieved from https://apps.who.int/iris/handle/10665/1871

[256] Rosengren, A., Smyth, A., Rangarajan, S, et al (2019). Socioeconomic Status and Risk of Cardiovascular Disease in 20 Low-income, Middle-income, and High-income Countries: The Prospective Urban Rural Epidemiologic (PURE) Study. Retrieved from https://www.thelancet.com/journals/langlo/article/PIIS2214-109X(19)30045-2/fulltext

[257] Mocumbi A. O. (2012). Lack of focus on cardiovascular disease in

sub-Saharan Africa. Cardiovascular diagnosis and therapy, 2(1), 74–77. https://doi.org/10.3978/j.issn.2223-3652.2012.01.03. Retrieved from https://www.ncbi.nlm.nih.gov/pmc/articles/PMC3839174/

[258] Antony KK. (1980). The pattern of cardiac failure in Northern Savanna Nigeria. Trop Geogr Med 1980;32:118-25.

[259] Oyoo GO, Ogola EN. Clinical and socio demographic aspects of congestive heart failure patients at Kenyatta National Hospital, Nairobi. East Afr Med J. 1999 Jan;76(1):23-7. PMID: 10442143.

[260] Shiel, Jr., William C. Asthma Rates Increasing . . . Are Environmental Exposures? Retrieved from https://medicinenet.com/asthma_rates_increasing/views.htm

[261] WHO Regional Committee for Africa. Cardiovascular diseases in the African region: current situation and perspectives-report of the regional director 2005. Retrieved from https://apps.who.int/iris/handle/10665/1871

[262] Rosengren, A., Smyth, A., Rangarajan, S, et al (2019). Socioeconomic Status and Risk of Cardiovascular Disease in 20 Low-income, Middle-income, and High-income Countries: The Prospective Urban Rural Epidemiologic (PURE) Study. Retrieved from https://www.thelancet.com/journals/langlo/article/PIIS2214-109X(19)30045-2/fulltext

[263] Colley JRT, Reid DD. Urban and social origins of childhood bronchitis in England and Wales. British Medical Journal, 1970, 2: 213–217.

[264]   Chronic Respiratory Diseases in Developing Countries: The Burden and Strategies for Prevention and Management Retrieved from https://www.who.int/bulletin/archives/79(10)971.pdf.

[265]   Global Burden of Disease Pediatrics Collaboration. Global and national burden of diseases and injuries among children and adolescents between 1990 and 2013; Retrieved from https://jamanetwork.com/journals/jamapediatrics/fullarticle/2481809

[266]   Zar, H.J., Vanker, A., Gray, D., and Zampoli, M. (2017). The African Pediatric Fellowship Training Program in Pediatric Pulmonology: A Model for Growing African Capacity in Child Lung Health. Retrieved from https://www.atsjournals.org/doi/full/10.1513/AnnalsATS.201612-953PS

[267]   Alberto Coustasse, Raghav Sarkar, Bukola Abodunde, Brandon J. Metzger, and Chelsea M. Slater.(2019). Use of Teledermatology to Improve Dermatological Access in Rural Areas . Telemedicine and e-Health. Nov 2019.1022-1032.http://doi.org/10.1089/tmj.2018.0130. Retrieved from https://www.liebertpub.com/doi/full/10.1089/tmj.2018.0130

[268]   Dermatologist Can Use Telemedicine Durig COVID-19 Outbreak. Retrieved from https://www.aad.org/member/practice/telederm/toolkit

[269]   Sreelatha, O. K., & Ramesh, S. V. (2016). Teleophthalmology: improving patient outcomes? Clinical ophthalmology (Auckland, N.Z.), 10,

285–295. https://doi.org/10.2147/OPTH.S80487. Retrieved from https://www.ncbi.nlm.nih.gov/pmc/articles/PMC4755429/

[270] Chapter 7: Teleophthalmology from Zhang A, & Yoon C.Y., & Zimmer-Galler I.E. (). Teleophthalmology. Rheuban K, & Krupinski E.A.(Eds.), Understanding Telehealth. McGraw-Hill. https://accessmedicine.mhmedical.com/content.aspx?bookid=2217&sectionid=187794772.

[271] Advances in Telemedicine in Ophthalmology. Prikh, D.; Armstrong, G.; Likou, V.; Husain, D. (2020). Seminars in Ophthalmology Vol. 35, 2020 Issue . Retrieved from https://www.tandfonline.com/doi/full/10.1080/08820538.2020.1789675

[272] Lea, Janice P. (2020).The Role of Telemedicine in Providing Nephrology Care in Rural Hospitals. Retrieved from https://kidney360.asnjournals.org/content/kidney360/early/2020/04/23/KID.0001122019.full.pdf

[273] Belcher, Justin M. (2020). The Role of Telenephrology in the Management of CKD. Retrieved from https://kidney360.asnjournals.org/content/1/11/1310

[274] Swee, Melissa L; Sanders, M. Lee, Phisitkul, Kantima, et al (2020). Development and Implementation of a Telenephrology Dashboard for Active Surveillance of Kidney Disease: A Quality Improvement Project. Retrieved from https://bmcnephrol.biomedcentral.com/articles/10.1186/s12882-020-02077-0

[275] Chronic Kidney Disease is Still a Major Heath challenge ihn Africa.

Retrieved from https://www.iol.co.za/lifestyle/health/chronic-kidney-disease-is-still-a-major-health-challenge-in-africa-11903844#:~:text=Chronic%20kidney%20disease%20is%20still%20a%20major%20health,failure%20and%20HIV.%20...%204%20Making%20changes.%20

[276] Kaze, A.D., Ilori, T., Jaar, B.G. et al. Burden of chronic kidney disease on the African continent: a systematic review and meta-analysis. BMC Nephrol 19, 125 (2018). https://doi.org/10.1186/s12882-018-0930-5. Retrieved from https://bmcnephrol.biomedcentral.com/articles/10.1186/s12882-018-0930-5

[277] Ganchimeg T, Ota E, Morisaki N, et al. Pregnancy and childbirth outcomes among adolescent mothers: A World Health Organization multicounty study. BJOG 2014;121 Suppl 1:40–8. Retrieved from https://obgyn.onlinelibrary.wiley.com/doi/full/10.1111/1471-0528.12630

[278] Althabe F, Moore JL, Gibbons L, et al. Adverse maternal and perinatal outcomes in adolescent pregnancies: The Global Network's Maternal Newborn Health Registry study. Reprod Health 2015;12 Suppl 2:S8. Retrieved from https://reproductive-health-journal.biomedcentral.com/articles/10.1186/1742-4755-12-S2-S8

[279] Maternal Mortality. Retrieved from https://www.who.int/news-room/fact-sheets/detail/maternal-mortality

[280] Telehealth Improves Obstetric and Gynecologic Health Outcomes. Retrieved from https://healthmanagement.org/c/it/news/telehealth-improves-obstetric-and-gynecologic-health-outcomes

[281] Implementing Telehealth in Practice, Obstetrics & Gynecology: February 2020 - Volume 135 - Issue 2 - p e73-e79 doi: 10.1097/AOG.0000000000003671. Retrieved from https://journals.lww.com/greenjournal/Fulltext/2020/02000/Implementing_Telehealth_in_Practice.44.aspx

[282] IARC Global Cancer Observatory, /https://www.cancerhealth.com/article/world-health-organization-releases-latest-global-cancer-data

[283] Infection Causes 1 in 6 Cancers Worldwide: Study. Retrieved from https://www.medicinenet.com/script/main/art.asp?articlekey=157956

[284] Cancer Care in Africa: An Overview of Resources. Retrieved from https://ascopubs.org/doi/full/10.1200/JGO.2015.000406

[285] Maserat, E. (2008). Information communication technology: new approach for rural cancer care improvement.\AsianPacJCancerPrev. Retrieved from https://scholar.google.com/citations?user=q1yk-KUoAAAAJ&hl=en#d=gs_md_cita-d&u=%2Fcitations%3Fview_op%3Dview_citation%26hl%3Den%26user%3Dq1ykKUoAAAAJ%26citation_for_view%3Dq1ykKUoAAAAJ%3AUeHWp8X0CEIC%26tzom%3

[286] Taking up Africa's cancer challenge. Retrieved from https://www.who.int/bulletin/volumes/96/4/18-020418/en/

[287] Stefan, Daniela Cristina, Cancer Care in Africa: An Overview of Resources. DOI: 10.1200/JGO.2015.000406 Journal of Global Oncology 1, no. 1 (October 01, 2015) 30-36. Retrieved from: https://ascopubs.org/

doi/full/10.1200/JGO.2015.000406

[288] The Financial Benefits of Telepathology. Retrieved from https://specialistdirectinc.com/telepathology-en/the-financial-benefits-of-telepathology/

[289] Telepathology. Retrieved from https://www.sciencedirect.com/topics/medicine-and-dentistry/telepathology

[290] United Nations Department of Economic and Social Affairs World Urbanization Prospects: the 2009 Revision Population Database. 2010. Retrieved from https://www.ipcc.ch/apps/njlite/ar5wg2/njlite_download2.php?id=10148

[291] World Health Organization. World health report 2006: working together for health. Geneva: WHO Press; 2006. Retrieved from https://www.who.int/whr/2006/en/

[292] United Nations Department of Economic Social Affairs Population Division, Retrieved from https://www.un.org/development/desa/pd/

[293] The Case for Telemedicine and Endocrinology; Retrieved from https://visuwell.io/telemedicine/endocrinology/

[294] World Health Organization. Atlas: Country Resources for Neurological Disorders. Geneva: World Health Organization; 2004. Retrieved from https://www.who.int/mental_health/neurology/epidemiology/en/

[295] Abdeslam El Khamlichi, M.D., African Neurosurgery: Current Situation, Priorities, and Needs, Neurosurgery, Volume 48, Issue 6, June 2001, Pages 1344-1347, https://doi.org/10.1097/00006123-200106000-00034

[296] El Khamlichi, A. (1998). African Neurosurgery Part II: Current State and Future Prospects; Surg Neurol. 1998 Mar;49(3):342-7. doi: 10.1016/s0090-3019(96)00423-5. PMID: 9508129.

[297] Hyder, A. A.; Wunderlich, C. A.; Puvanachandra, P., et al; (2007). The Impact of Traumatic Brain Injuries: A Global Perspective. Neuro. Rehabil., 22 (2007), pp. 341-353/

[298] Africa's Neurologist Shortage 30 Aug 2019. Retrieved from https://wfneurology.org/africas-neurologist-shortage

[299] The Haitian Foundation for the Development of Neurology and Neurosurgery. Retrieved from: https://fhadnneceng.WordPress.com/

[300] The rise of neurology in Haiti. Retrieved from: https://www.thelancet.com/journals/laneur/article/PIIS1474-4422(18)30431-9/fulltext

[301] Ensuring an Adequate Neurosurgical Workforce or the 21st Century: A Statement of the American Association of Neurological Surgeons, American Board of Neurological Surgery, Congress of Neurological Surgeons, Society of Neurological Surgeons. (2012). Retrieved from: https://www.aans.org/pdf/Legislative/Neurosurgery%20IOM%20GME%20Paper%2012%2019%2012.pdf

[302] Kenning, Tyler J., MD, FAANS (2016). Neurosurgical Workforce Shortage: The Effect of Sub specialization and a Case or Shortening Residency Training. Retrieved from: https://aansneurosurgeon.org/departments/neurosurgical-workforce-shortage-effect-subspecialization-cast-shortening-residency-training/

[303] Center for Workforce Studies. (2012). Physician specialty datebook. Retrieved from https://www.aamc.org/system/files/reports/1/2012physicianspecialtydatabook.pdf

[304] World Health Organization (WHO) World Health Statistics 2008. Geneva: WHO; 2008). Retrieved from: http://www.who.int/whosis/whostat/`2008/en/index.html

[305] World Health Organization (WHO) World Health Report 2006: working together for health. Geneva: WHO; 2006. Retrieved from: URL: https://www.who.int/whr/2006/en/

[306] Task Force for Scaling Up Education and Training for Health Workers, Global Health Workforce Alliance. Scaling up, saving lives. Geneva: Global Health Workforce Alliance; 2008. Retrieved from https://www.who.int/workforcealliance/documents/Global_Health%20FINAL%20REPORT.pdf

[307] Kwon, Y. S.; Tabakin, A. L.; Patel, H. V; et al (2020). Adapting Urology Residency Training in the COVID-19 Era. Retrieved from https://goldjournal.net/article/50090-4295(20)30452-0/fulltext.

[308]   Gettman, M.; Rhee, E; and Spitz, A. (2016). Telemedicine in Urology. White Paper, The American Urological Association. Retrieved from https://auanet.org/guidelines/telemedicine-in-urology

[309]   Hagander L.E., Hughes C.D., Nash K., Ganjawalla K., Linden A., Martins Y. Surgeon migration between developing countries and the United States: train, retain, and gain from brain drain. World J Surg. 2013.

[310]   Murray CJ, Vos T, Lozano R, Naghavi M, Flaxman AD, Michaud C, et al. Disability-adjusted life years (DALYs) for 291 diseases and injuries in 21 regions, 1990-2010: a systematic analysis for the Global Burden of Disease Study 2010. Lancet. 2012; 380:2197–223.

[311]   Vos T, Flaxman AD, Naghavi M, Lozano R, Michaud C, Ezzati M, et al. Years lived with disability (YLDs) for 1160 sequelae of 289 diseases and injuries 1990-2010: a systematic analysis for the Global Burden of Disease Study 2010. Lancet. 2012;380:2163–96.

[312]   Mody, G.M. Rheumatology in Africa—challenges and opportunities. Arthritis Res Ther 19, 49 (2017). https://doi.org/10.1186/s13075-017-1259-3 https://arthritis-research.biomedcentral.com/articles/10.1186/s13075-017-1259-3

[313]   Nabalamba, A., Chikoko, M. (2011). Aging Population Changes in Africa. AfDB Chief Economist Complex,Vol1. Issue 1, November 2011.

[314]   Population ages 65 and above for the Virgin Islands of the United States; ALFRED Archival Economic Data.

[315]　　Population Pyramids of the World from1950 to2100 retrieved from https://populationpyramid.net/haiti/2030

[316]　　https://healthequityintl.org/our-work/non-infectious-diseases

[317]　　Maternal Mortality; The World Health Organization; retrieved from https://who.int/news-room/fact-sheets/detail/maternal-mortality

[318]　　WHO. Women and Health. Today's Evidence, Tomorrow's Agenda. http://whqlibdoc.who.int/publications/2009/9789241563857_eng.pdf

[319]　　WHO, UNICEF, UNFPA, The World Bank. Trends in maternal mortality: 1990 to 2008. Retrieved from https://www.unfpa.org/featured-publication/trends-maternal-mortality-2000-2017

[320]　　World Health Organization. Neonatal and Perinatal Mortality. Country, Regional and Global Estimates. Geneva, Switzerland: World Health Organization; 2006. Retrieved from https://apps.who.int/iris/handle/10665/43444

[321]　　Global health workforce shortage to reach 12.9 million in coming decades. Retrieved from https://www.who.int/mediacentre/news/releases/2013/health-workforce-shortage/en/

[322]　　Zurn P, Dolea C, Stilwell B. Nurse retention and recruitment: developing a motivated workforce. Genva: International Council of Nurses; 2005. Retrieved from https://www.researchgate.net/publication/253159418_Nurse_Retention_and_Recruitment_Develop-

ing_a_Motivated_Workforce

[323] Mullan F. The metrics of the physician brain drain. N Engl J Med 2005; 353:1810-1818 DOI: 10.1056/NEJMsa050004. Retrieved from https://www.nejm.org/doi/full/10.1056/NEJMsa050004

[324] Global Shortage of Health Workers and its Impact; retrieved from: http://globalhealthlearning.org/sites/default/files/page-files/Global_Shortage_of_Health_Workers.pdf

[325] EVA for Teleconsultation. https://mobileodt.com/solutions/tele-consultation/?doing_wp_cron=1608849289.0625920295715332031250

[326] Lowery, C.; (2018). Telehealth: A New Frontier for Ob/Gyn. Retrieved from https://contemporaryobgyn.net/view/telehealth-new-frontier-obgyn

[327] http://phb.secondsensehearing.com/content/which-country-has-most-hearing-loss;

[328] Desalew, A.; Gelano, T.F; Semahegn, A., et al (2020). Childhood Hearing Impairment and its Associated Factors in Sub-Saharan Africa in the 21st Century: A Systematic Review and Meta-Analysis. Retrieved from https://www.ncbi.nlm.nih.gov/pmc/articles/PMC7222652/

[329] WHO Childhood Hearing Loss: Act Now, Here's How. Retrieved from https://www.who.int/pbd/deafness/world-hearing-day/WHD2016_Brochure_EN_2.pdf

[330]   Causes of Hearing Loss in Africa. Retrieved from: https://www.hear-it.org/causes-of-hearing-loss-in-africa

[331]   Olusanya BO, Neumann KJ, Saunders JE. The global burden of disabling hearing impairment: a call to action. Bulletin of the World Health Organization. 2014; 92(5): 367-73. /

[332]   WHO estimates (2002) https://www.who.int/pbd/deafness/facts/en//

[333]   https://www.who.int/pbd/deafness/hearing_impairment_grades/en/

[334]   Audiology Service Delivery considerations in Health Care During COID-10. Retrieved from: https://www.asha.org/aud/Audiology-Service-Delivery-Considerations-in-Health-Care-During-Coronavirus-COVID-19/

[335]   Clinical governance and Teleaudiology. Retrieved from: https://hearinghealthmatters.org/innovationsinhearing/2019/clinical-governance-teleaudiology/

[336]   Clinical governance and Teleaudiology Retrieved from: https://hearinghealthmatters.org/innovationsinhearing/2019/clinical-governance-teleaudiology/

[337]   Current Practices in Tele-audiology Retrieved from: https://www.audiology.org/practice_management/resources/current-practices-tele-audiology

[338] Haiti: On the Road to Sustainability; retrieved from: https://www.hearingreview.com/practice-building/practice-management/continuing-education/hear-haiti-road-sustainability#:~:text=A%20Shelter%20of%20Hope%20for%20People%20with%20Hearing,than%20160%20deaf%20families%20established%20a%20community%20here.

[339] New Generation of Cochlear Implants – New Face of Telemedicine. Retrieved from https://whc.ifps.org.pl/en/2018/12/next-generation-of-cochlear-implants-a-new-face-of-telemedicine/

[340] Lewis TL, Wyatt JC. mHealth and mobile medical apps: a framework to assess risk and promote safer use. J Med Internet Res. 2014. Retrieved from: https://www.jmir.org/2014/9/e210/

[341] Thornton, D., Brinkhuis, M., Amrit, C. & Aly, R. 2015. 'Categorizing and describing the types of fraud in healthcare', Procedia Computer Science, 64:713-720. Retrieved from: https://www.sciencedirect.com/science/article/pii/S1877050915027295

[342] Garuba HA, Kohler JC, Huisman AM. Transparency in Nigeria's public pharmaceutical sector: perceptions from policymakers. Global Health. 2009; 5:14. doi: 10.1186/1744-8603-5-14. Retrieved from: https://globalizationandhealth.biomedcentral.com/articles/10.1186/1744-8603-5-14

[343] Cohen JC, Mrazek M, Hawkins L. Tackling corruption in the pharmaceutical systems worldwide with courage and conviction. Clin Pharmacol Ther. 2007; 81:445-449. doi: 10.1038/sj.clpt.6100074. Retrieved from http://www.g8.utoronto.ca/conferences/2010/ghdp/

cohen-mrazek-hawkins-corruption.pdf

[344] USA Shappert Announces Launch of V.I. Health Care Fraud Task Force. Retrieved from https://www.justice.gov/usao-vi/pr/usa-shappert-announces-launch-vi-health-care-fraud-task-force

[345] Corruption in Sub-Saharan Africa. Retrieved at https://www.cfr.org/backgrounder/corruption-sub-saharan-africa

[346] Upholding the fight against corruption in the Caribbean https://thecommonwealth.org/media/news/upholding-fight-against-corruption-caribbean

[347] An Anatomy of Corruption: Haiti. Retrieved from https://www.csis.org/analysis/anatomy-corruption-haiti;

[348] Building Corruption in Haiti. Retrieved from https://nacla.org/news/2019/10/03/corruption-haiti-petrocaribe

[349] 5 Facts About Health Care in Haiti. Retrieved from https://borgenproject.org/5-facts-about-health-care-in-haiti/

[350] Corruption. Retrieved from https://www.globalsecurity.org/military/world/haiti/corruption.htm

[351] Fighting Corruption in the Health Sector: Methods, Tools, and Good Practices. https://anti-corruption.org/wp-content/uploads/2017/05/Anticorruption-Methods-and-Tools-in-Health-Lo-Res-final-1.pdf

[352]   https://www.worldometers.info/coronavirus/

[353]   https://www.who.int/emergencies/diseases/novel-coronavirus-2019

[354]   https://www.msn.com/en-us/news/coronavirus?ocid=spartandhp

[355]   Telehealth in Rural Communities. Retrieved from: https://www.cdc.gov/chronicdisease/resources/publications/factsheets/tele-health-in-rural-communities.htm

APPENDIX C:
OTHER WORKS RESEARCHED IN THE WRITING OF THIS BOOK

1. Marc H, Byong-Joon K, editors. Building Good Governance: Reforms in Seoul. National Center for Public Productivity; 2002.

2. Barro R. Democracy and Growth. Journal of Economic Growth. 1996;1:1-27.

3. United Nations Development Programme, author. Governance for sustainable human development, UNDP policy document. New York: 1997.

4. https://www.ncbi.nlm.nih.gov/pmc/articles/PMC3092326/.

5. Wilkinson R, Pickett K. Income Inequality and Social Dysfunction. Annu Rev Social. 2009;35:493-511.

6. Collier P. The bottom billion: why the poorest countries are failing

and what can be done about it. Oxford University Press: 2007.

7. United Nations Development Programme, author. Governance for sustainable human development, UNDP policy document. New York: 1997.

8. https://www.theatlantic.com/politics/archive/2017/08/what-health-reform-means-to-the-american-territories/538056/

9. WHO, New Report on Corruption; retrieved from

10. https://www.transparency.org/en/our-priorities/health-and-corruption

11. https://www.vi.gov/healthier-horizons/

12. http://www.virginislandsdailynews.com/business/plessen-pioneers-telemedicine-in-the-usvi/article_343b3a0f-fa1d-5baa-9ade-34c1280c3048.html

13. https://www.ncbi.nlm.nih.gov/pmc/articles/PMC5206488/pdf/nihms835996.pdf

14. https://www2.deloitte.com/us/en/insights/industry/public-sector/virtual-health-telemedicine-rural-areas.html

15. A health telematics policy in support of WHO's Health-For-All strategy for global health development: report of the WHO group consultation on health telematics, 11–16 December, Geneva, 1997. Geneva,

World Health Organization, 1998. Retrieved from https://apps.who.int/iris/handle/10665/63857

16. State of Health Financing in the African Region, January 2013. Retrieved from https://www.afro.who.int/sites/default/files/2017-06/state-of-health-financing-afro.pdf

17. Blewett LA, Call KT, Marmor S. Health reform and the US Virgin Islands: high-need-limited impact. J Public Health Manag Pract. 2013 Sep-Oct;19(5):393-401. doi: 10.1097/PHH.0b013e31826d8020. PMID: 23446878.

18. Baum, N.; Kikrshenbaum, E.; Rhee, E.Y. (2019). Teleurology: The Time has Arrived. Urology Times Journal, Vol. 47 No 10, Volume 47, Issue 10; Retrieved from Https://urologytimes.com/view/teleurology-time-has-arrived.

19. Tele-urology moves from concept to practice; retrieved from https://urologytimes.com/view/tele-urology-moves-concept-practice

20. Koraishy, F. M., Rohatgi, R. (2020). Telenephrology: An Emerging Platform for Delivering Renal Health Care; American Journal of Kidney Diseases (AJKD), June 02, 2020; DOI:https://doi.org/10.1053/j.ajkd.2020.02.442.

21. Implementing Telehealth in Practice, Obstetrics & Gynecology: February 2020 - Volume 135 - Issue 2 - p e73-e79 doi: 10.1097/AOG.0000000000003671

22. Moore, K., (2017). Teleaudiology 101. Retrieved from: https://www.audiologyonline.com/articles/teleaudiology-101-19711

23. Coco, L. (2020). Teleaudiology: Strategies, Considerations During a Crisis and Beyond. The Hearing Journal: May 2020 - Volume 73 - Issue 5 - p 26,28,29 doi: 10.1097/01.HJ.0000666404.42257.97. Retrieved from: https://journals.lww.com/thehearingjournal/fulltext/2020/05000/teleaudiology__strategies,_considerations_during_a.3.aspx

24. Hearing Loss in Africa. Retrieved from: https://www.hear-it.org/hearing-loss-in-africa

25. Causes of Hearing Loss in Africa. Retrieved from: https://www.hear-it.org/causes-of-hearing-loss-in-africa

26. Bulletin of the World Health Organization. Policy & Practice. The Global Burden of Disabling Hearing Impairment: A Call to Action. Retrieved from: https://www.who.int/bulletin/volumes/92/5/13-128728/en/

27. Moffatt, Jennifer & Eley, Diann S. (2011). Barriers to the up-take of telemedicine in Australia – a view from providers. Retrieved from https://www.rrh.org.au/journal/article/1581

28. Baldoni, S., Amenta, F., & Ricci, G. (2019). Telepharmacy Services: Present Status and Future Perspectives: A Review. Medicina (Kaunas, Lithuania), 55(7), 327. https://doi.org/10.3390/medicina55070327

29. Desalew, A., Feto Gelano, T., Semahegn, A., Geda, B., & Ali, T.

(2020). Childhood hearing impairment and its associated factors in sub-Saharan Africa in the 21st century: A systematic review and meta-analysis. SAGE open medicine, 8, 2050312120919240. https://doi.org/10.1177/2050312120919240

30. Which Country has the Most Hearing Loss? Retrieved from: http://phb.secondsensehearing.com/content/which-country-has-most-hearing-loss

31. Juvet, T.; Hayes, J.R.; Ferrara, S.; et al. (2020). The Burden of Urological Disease in Zomba, Malawi: A Needs Assessment in a Sub-Saharan Tertiary Care Center. Can Urol Assoc J 2020; 14(1):E6-12. http://dx.doi.org/10.5489/cuaj.5837. Retrieved from: https://www.ncbi.nlm.nih.gov/pmc/articles/PMC6955180/pdf/cuaj-1-e6.pdf

32. Miseda, M. H.; Were, S.O.; Murianki, C.A.; (2017). The Implication of the Shortage of Health Workforce Specialist on Universal Coverage in Kenya. Hum Resour Health 15, 80 (2017). https://doi.org/10.1186/s12960-017-0253-9. Retrieved from: https://human-resources-health.biomedcentral.com/articles/10.1186/s12960-017-0253-9

33. Shortage of Doctors is Beyond Critical (2011). Mail & Guardian. Retrieved from: https://mg.co.za/article/2011-08-05-shortage-of-doctors-is-beyond-critical/

34. Loughlin, K. R. (2018). Addressing the Urology Doctor Shortage: Implications for Patient Care. Harvard Medical School, Lean Forward. Retrieved from: https://leanforward.hms.harvard.edu/2019/02/14/

addressing-the-urology-doctor-shortage-implications-for-patient-care/

35. Tele-Urology: Access and Quality of Care for Patients. The American Urological Association. Retrieved from: https://www.disabled-world.com/medical/ehealth/Teleurology.php

36. Sylora, J. A. (2019). Telehealth in Urology Presented during the 29th Annual International Prostate Cancer Update on January 25,2019 in Beaver Creek, Colorado. Retrieved from: https://grandroundsinurology.com/tele-health-in-urology/

37. (2016) Tele-Urology Improves Access and Quality of Care for Patients. Retrieved from https://www.prnewswire.com/news-releases/tele-urology-improves-access-and-quality-of-care-for-patients-300264192.html#:~:text=Within%20the%20urologic%20community%2C%20tele-medicine%2C%20also%20referred%20to,postoperative%20care%2C%20second%20opinions%20and%2C%20possibly%2C%20remote%20surgery.

38. Tele-Urology versus Face-to-Face Clinics: A Survey of Patient Preference. Journal of Urology Vol. 195,No.45, Supplement, Saturday, May 7, 2016, MP31-07. Retrieved from https://www.auajournals.org/doi/pdf/10.1016/j.juro.2016.02.1260

39. Schladetzky, Z. (2018). The 4 Different Types of Telepharmacy. Retrieved from: https://blog.telepharm.com/the-4-different-types-of-telepharmacy

40. Graham LE, Zimmerman M, Vassallo DJ, et al. Telemedicine--the way

ahead for medicine in the developing world. Trop Doct. 2003; 33:36–8.

41. Government of Uganda, ministry of health, national health policy: Reducing poverty through promoting people's health. 2009 May; Version.

42. Ganapathy K. Telemedicine and neurosciences in developing countries. Surg Neurol. 2002; 58:388–94.

43. Oberholzer M, Christen H, Haroske G, et al. Modern telepathology: a distributed system with open standards. Curr Probl Dermatol. 2003; 32:102–14.

44. Wright D. Telemedicine and developing countries. A report of study group 2 of the ITU Development Sector. J Telemed Telecare. 1998;4(Suppl 2):1–85.

45. Kenyan ICT Health Conference calls for a National Telemedicine Centre. [Last accessed on 2013 Mar 06]. Available from: http://www.aitecafrica.com

46. Adeyinka MB. Fundamentals of modern telemedicine in Africa. Methods Inf Med. 1997; 36:95–8.

47. Pan African e-network Project. Inauguration of Pan-African e-Network Project (Phase 2) TCIL Bhawan, New Delhi on 16 th August 2010

48. Telemedicine. Khartoum-Sudan. http://www.ashracom.net/telcom

49. Nzeyimana D. Assessment of telemedicine in Rwanda, current and future State. 2012

50. Africa Renewal (2010), For African business, ending corruption is 'priority number one', published by United Nations Africa Renewal, New York, NY 10017 USA

51. Claire, F. (2010), Corruption in Africa: A Crime against Development, retrieved January 24, 2015.

52. The Guardian (2010), Corruption Index 2010 from Transparency International: find out how each Country Compares, retrieved January 22, 2015.

53. Transparency International (2015), Corruption in Africa: 75 Million People Pay Bribes, Published November 30, 2015

54. United Nations Millennium Development Goals Report, New York, United Nations, retrieved January 24, 2015.

55. Zurn P, Dolea C, Stilwell B. Nurse retention and recruitment: developing a motivated workforce [Issue paper 4]. Geneva: International Council of Nurses; 2005. Available from: http://www.icn.ch/global/Issue4Retention.pdf [accessed on 23 January 2009].

56. Mullan F. The metrics of the physician brain drain. N Engl J Med 2005; 353: 1810-8 doi: 10.1056/NEJMsa050004 pmid: 16251537.

57. Leibbrandt M, Woolard I, Finn A, et al. Trends in South African Income Distribution and Poverty since the Fall of Apartheid. OECD Social, Employment and Migration. Working Papers, No. 101. Paris: OECD Publishing, 2010. http://dx.doi.org/10.1787/5kmms0t7p1ms-en

58. World Health Organization. Closing the Gap in a Generation. Health Equity through Action on the Social Determinants of Health. Geneva: World Health Organization. http://www.who.int/social_determinants/thecommission/finalreport/en/index.html (accessed 30 December 2012).

59. Birn A-E. Addressing the Societal Determinants of Health: The key Global Health Ethics imperative. In: Benatar S, Brock G, eds. Global Health and Global Health Ethics. Cambridge: Cambridge University Press, 2011:37-52.

60. Relman AS. Medical professionalism in a commercialized health care market. JAMA 2007; 298:2668-2670.

61. Benatar SR, Gill S, Bakker IC. Global health and the global economic crisis. Am J Public Health 2011;101(4):646-653.

62. As, I.H. (2002). Learning in organizations working with telemedicine. Journal of Telemedicine & Telecare, 8, 107-111.

63. Dusserre, L., Retaillau, B., & Cotran, P. (1996). Evaluation of an international telepathology system between Boston (USA) and Dijon: glass slides versus telediagnostic television monitor. Journal of Telemedicine

& Telecare, 2, 27-30.

64. Bartholmai, B.J., Erickson, B.J., Hartman, T.E., King, B.F., Meredith-James, E., Hangiandreou, N.J., & Williamson, B. (2002). The electronic imaging technology specialist: the role of a new radiology subspecialty for the 21st century. Journal of Digital Imaging, 15, 184-188.

65. A., Cobelli, C., Nucci, G., Del Prato, S., Maran, A., Kilkki, E., & Tuominen, J. (2002). A telemedicine support for diabetes management: The T-IDDM project. Computer Methods & Programs in Biomedicine, 69, 147-161.

66. Chen, K., Lim, A., & Shumack, S. (2002). Teledermatology: influence of zoning and education on a clinician's ability to observe peripheral lesions. Australasian Journal of Dermatology, 43, 171-174.

67. Della-Mea, V., Cortolezzis, D., & Beltrami, C.A. (2000). The economics of telepathology--a case study. Journal of Telemedicine & Telecare, 6, 168-169.

68. Telepathology using internet multimedia electronic mail: remote consultation on gastrointestinal pathology. Journal of Telemedicine & Telecare, 2, 38-34.

69. Doarn, C.R., Fitzgerald, S., Rodas, E., Harnett, B., Prabe- Egge, A., & Merrell, R.C. (2002). Telemedicine to integrate intermittent surgical services into primary care. Telemedicine Journal & E-Health, 8, 131-137.

70. Drozdov, D.V., Obukhova, E.O., Orlov, O.I., Levanov, V.M., Nenast'eva, O.K., & Sergeev. D.V. (2002). Introduction of telemedical electrocardiographic system in regional hospital. Klinicheskaia Meditsina, 80, 62-66.

71. Field, M.J. (1996). Telemedicine: A guide to assessing telecommunications in health care. Washington, D.C.: Institute of Medicine.

72. Goldenberg, D., & Wenig, B.L. (2002). Telemedicine in otolaryngology. American Journal of Otolaryngology, 23, 35-43.

73. Gombas, P., Skepper, J.N., & Hegyi, L. (2002). The image pyramid system--an unbiased, inexpensive and broadly accessible method of telepathology.

74. Telemedicine as a tool for intensive management of diabetes: the DIABTel experience. Computer Methods & Programs in Biomedicine, 69, 163-177.

75. Hilty, D.M., Luo, J.S., Morache, C., Marcelo, D.A., & Nesbitt, T.S. (2002). Telepsychiatry: an overview for psychiatrists. CNS Drugs, 16, 527-548.

76. Jukic, D.M., & Bifulco, C.B. (1999). Telepathology and pathology at distance: an overview. Croatian Medical Journal, 40, 421-424.

77. Krupinski, E., Barker, G., Rodriquez, G., Engstrom, M., Levine, N., Lopez, A.M., & Weinstein, R.S. (2002). Telemedicine versus in-person dermatology referrals: an analysis of case complexity. Telemedicine Journal and E-Health, 8, 143-147.

78. Lim, A.C., Egerton, I.B., See, A., & Schumack, S.P. (2001). Accuracy and reliability of store-and-forward Teledermatology: preliminary results from the St George Teledermatology Project. Australasian Journal of Dermatology, 42, 247-251.

79. Linderoth, H.C. (2002). Managing telemedicine: from noble ideas to action. Journal of Telemedicine & Telecare, 8, 143-150.

80. Maheu, M.M., Whitten, P., & Allen, A. (2001). Ehealth, telehealth, and telemedicine: A guide to start-up and success (1st ed.). Danvers, MA: Jossey-Bass.

81. Mairinger, T. (2000). Acceptance of telepathology in daily practice. Analytical Cellular Pathology, 21, 135-140.

82. Miller, G.G., & Levesque, K. (2002). Telehealth provides effective pediatric surgery care to remote locations. Journal of Pediatric Surgery, 37, 752-754.

83. Sable, C. (2002). Digital echocardiology and telemedicine applications in pediatric cardiology. Pediatric Cardiology, 23, 358-369.

84. Williams, B.H., Mullick, F.G., Butler, D.R., Herring, R.F., & O'leary, T.J. (2001). Clinical evaluation of an international static image-based telepathology service. Human Pathology, 32, 1309-1317.

85. Yadav, H., & Lin, W.Y. (2001). Patient confidentiality, ethics, and licensing in telemedicine. Asia-Pacific Journal of Public Health, 13, 36-38.

APPENDIX D:
ALSO BY DR. HUGUES FIDELE BATSIELILIT PHD

False-Positive HIV Test Results: The Silent Issue in African Countries

This book is written as a result of the findings and experiences of Dr. Hugues Fidele Batsielilit, Ph.D., during the implementation of infectious diseases programs in several African countries. Sadly, he observed there was consistent denial of existing evidence of false-positive HIV test results within African communities, particularly in areas of underprivileged populations living in remote areas.

The writing of this book was further prompted by the disregard for the increasing impact false-positive results have on individuals and communities resulting in an overall failure in the confidence Africans have for battling the soaring negative impacts of HIV.

The issue of false-positive HIV test results should not be restricted to only perceptive or conceptual fact and advice for conventional harmless procedures. Rather, it must be presented and focused upon as a persistent and challenging negative issue with need for urgent actions along with diverse approaches to mitigate it and the pervasive impact it has on Africans.

This book can be purchased on Amazon by using this link https://www.amazon.com/False-Positive-HIV-Test-Results-Countries/dp/1480991171

APPENDIX E:
DON'T MISS OUT!

Dr. Hugues Fidele Batsielilit, Ph.D. is an avid writer and researcher. You do not want to miss out on any his new material, so please go to the link provided below to sign up for notifications whenever he publishes new content. There is no charge or obligation for doing so.

https://www.internationalconsultingaidnetwork.org/

www.ingramcontent.com/pod-product-compliance
Lightning Source LLC
Chambersburg PA
CBHW070619220526
45466CB00001B/60